CHILDREN

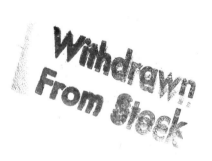

CHILDREN
AND
SPORT

FITNESS, INJURIES AND DIET

VIVIAN GRISOGONO

with contributions from
Jane Griffin and Craig Sharp

JOHN MURRAY

For Andrew

First published in 1991
by John Murray (Publishers) Ltd
50 Albemarle Street, London W1X 4BD

Paperback edition 1994

British Library Cataloguing-in-Publication Data

Grisogono, Vivian
   Children and sport.
   I. Title
   796.083

   ISBN 0–7195–4908–6

Typeset by Wearside Tradespools, Fulwell, Sunderland
Printed in Great Britain by Butler & Tanner Ltd, Frome & London

Contents

Acknowledgements   viii
Introduction   ix

I Background Factors   I

Definition of children and sport   1
Why do children take up sports?   2
Why do we worry?   7
Parents – oppressive or supportive?   10

2 Body Conditioning and Fitness Training   22

Selection of games and sports   22
Posture   25
Fitness training   26

3 The Exercise Physiology of Children
by Craig Sharp   32

The skeleton and general growth   33
Size, the growth spurt and puberty   35
Fat   37
Muscle strength   41
Muscle endurance (anaerobic fitness)   44
Aerobic fitness   47
Flexibility and mobility   61
Muscle versatility   66

Body temperature control   66
Dehydration   69
The child's view of exercise   69
Conclusions   70

4 Children's Pains and Injuries   72

'Growing pains'   72
'Clicking' joints   72
The need for diagnosis   73
How widespread are children's injuries?   74
Monitoring: the elite boys' squash squads   76
Possible after-effects and long-term risks of injuries   78
How to deal with children's pains and injuries   79

5 Why Do Children Get Injured?   82

6 Injury Prevention   94

Monitoring and measurements   96
Basic biomechanical tests (and remedial exercises)   100
Checklist for injury prevention   114

7 Bone Injuries   116

Traumatic fractures   118
Stress fractures   122
Apophysitis   126
Bone conditions and diseases   130

8 Soft-Tissue Injuries   132

The foot and leg   134
The thigh   140
The inner thigh, groin and hip   143
The trunk   144
The shoulder, arm and hand   148

9 Knee Injuries 152

Knee swelling 152
Cartilage tears 153
Cruciate ligament injuries 154
Medial ligament injuries 155
Dislocation 155
Patella alta 156
Fat pad impingement 156
Plica 157
Patellar tendon injuries 157
Knee-cap pain syndrome 158
Knee-cap subluxation and dislocation 163

10 Injury Case Studies 164

11 Diet for Children
by Jane Griffin 175

The importance of a balanced diet 176
Pre-school children 178
Hyperactivity 182
Food intolerance 183
School-age children 184
Teenagers 187
Anorexia nervosa and bulimia nervosa 195
Sports nutrition for children 196
Useful addresses 209

12 Conclusions 210

References 214

Index 232

Acknowledgements

For their help with various aspects of this book, I would like to thank Mrs Pat Grant of the Postgraduate Medical Centre, Ashford Hospital, Middlesex; Heather Medcalf and Ann Williams of the Birmingham University Documentation Centre for Sport; Mr John King, orthopaedic surgeon, and Dr David Perry, consultant rheumatologist, of the London Hospital; Gavin Bones; Daniel and Jessica Brogan; Matthew East; Sandy, Katie and Rory Farquharson; Alastair Fentiman; Sanil and Pooja Gautama; Lydia Haas; Saskia Stevenson; Mark, Lucy and Adam Thornby. I also have to thank the many kind parents who have allowed their children to contribute to the book.

Special thanks are owed to my good friends Jane Griffin and Craig Sharp for their patient efforts in producing expert specialist chapters; to Michael Bartlett for his superb artwork; and to Roger Hudson, long-suffering and ever-patient editor, whose expertise has shaped the book into coherent form.

Vivian Grisogono
Author

It is a pleasure to record my gratitude for the charming and competent help enthusiastically given by Heather Medcalf, Director of the Documentation Centre for Sport in the library of the University of Birmingham, and her assistant, Ann Williams. I would also like to thank my son Duncan very warmly for his effort, enthusiasm, motivation and patience during photography in the laboratories of the British Olympic Medical Centre.

Dr Craig Sharp
Contributor

Introduction

Children and sport are a controversial and much-discussed topic. There is often much argument, and little fact. Children themselves usually cannot contribute to the debate, as they lack the experience, and can only reflect the opinions of those influencing them. People involved in, or responsible for, children's sport, whether parents, sports coaches or schoolteachers, tend to have fixed opinions or uncertainties on which goals to aim for, and how best to achieve them. Most people agree, however, that children's participation in competitive sports can give rise to ethical, emotional, psychological, medical and physical problems, especially if the child specializes in a single sport from a young age. The ethical side, particularly, has become a subject for concern.[1] Serious competition inevitably requires the participant to be 'dedicated' and 'hard-working', although the effort can also bring great pleasure and delight.

Increasingly, medical, paramedical and scientific specialists are becoming involved in children's sport, on both practical and theoretical levels. Doctors, surgeons, physiotherapists, physiologists, dieticians and psychologists might all have a contribution to make towards ensuring that children participate in sport effectively and safely. Scientific research is being carried out world-wide on different aspects of children's sport, and is beginning to supply some definitions in place of prejudices and suppositions. The accumulation of repeatable scientific data to provide objective evidence is a painstaking process. Some of the questions seem unanswerable. As with other aspects of human activity and behaviour, one can only learn by observing individual achievements and responses.

Many people only consider the problems relating to children involved in 'serious' competitive sports. However, there are several areas of interest and concern beyond this, including the role of sport in promoting good body posture; sport as exercise for providing health and well-being; sport as a factor in disease prevention (especially heart disease); sport to help control medical conditions like asthma; and sport for disabled children. The relationship between children and sport is two-way, involving the suitability of the child for sport, and the relevance of sport to the child.

The main questions relating to children's sport tend to be:

1. What benefits, if any, can a child derive from sport?
2. Should children be taught the relationship between sport and exercise? If so, at what age?
3. Which sports are best for children? Are some sports bad for children?
4. Should new sports, or new versions of old sports, be designed for children?
5. How old should a child be before participating in organized sport and learning specific skills?
6. How much sport can or should a child be encouraged to do?
7. How competitive should children's sport be?
8. How soon, if at all, should a child specialize in a sport?
9. How much can a child be expected to achieve in learning the skills of a given sport?
10. What is the relationship between children's and adults' sports?
11. Can one predict later or adult success from childhood talent?
12. Should childhood sporting talent be sought out, simply allowed to emerge, or just ignored?
13. Should adults try to nurture a child's talent? If so, how best can they do so?
14. How does sports participation affect a child's relationships with adults and other children?
15. How does sports participation relate to a child's schooling and academic development?
16. Can competitive sport cause children emotional or psychological harm?
17. Do sporting children need special diets?
18. What are the physiological factors relevant to children's sport?
19. What medical problems can arise through children's sport?
20. What short- and long-term injury risks exist in children's sports?

In this book, we try to provide possible answers to those questions which pertain to an able-bodied, healthy child's physical development and well-being. We describe the various aspects of the subject that we deem the most important, from physiological, nutritional, and therapeutic standpoints, in order to identify problems and suggest possible approaches to them. We outline the current relevant research trends, and provide suggestions of worthwhile papers and books for further reading. Most importantly, we set out programmes for making children fitter and healthier, both *for* sport and *through* sport.

Our major aim is to present practical guidelines for making children's sport safe, effective, enjoyable and worthwhile. Our suggestions are only partly based on our reading and researches. They derive mainly from our practical experiences in dealing with sporting children, observing their successes, failures and problems, and helping them to achieve their best aspirations and to conquer their setbacks.

1 Background factors

Definition of children and sport

As our concern is the child's development, we are considering children from the youngest age, as babies, through to the end of their teenage years, when most of the major bone growth and body development processes are complete. Roughly speaking, we have taken 19 years as our upper age limit, so we cover both childhood and adolescence. We have to emphasize that age is not the sole criterion for judging the phases of growth and development. Individuals may mature relatively quickly or slowly, so, although we may refer to age-groups, particularly *pre-teen* and *teenage*, these are only guidelines as to the periods of development we are describing. Where we refer to 'very young children', this means roughly under the age of 7; 'young children' are under 11 years, and 'older children' are teenagers. Puberty is an important landmark in children's development, so in many instances we refer to three groups: pre-pubescent or pre-pubertal (before puberty, usually meaning younger than teenage); pubescent or pubertal (at the stage of puberty, which usually happens in the early teens); and post-pubescent or post-pubertal (after puberty, usually meaning mid to late teenage).

Play is the very essence of childhood, providing pleasure and entertainment. Many children's games are based on physical activity, and provide an outlet for surplus energy. It will be no surprise to parents that research on children's muscles has shown that they do not get tired easily![1] There is a close relationship between sports and games. Some definitions try to separate sports from games, others identify them as interchangeable.[2]

Our definition of sport, for the purposes of this book, is: a structured activity involving skills, movement, co-ordination, and an

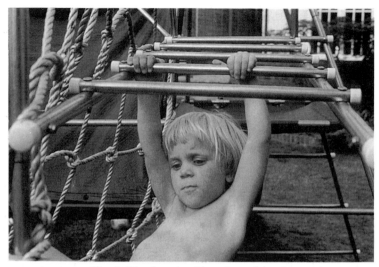

The climbing frame combines play and exercise.

appropriate level of physical fitness. There may be rules or laws governing the conduct of the participants. A sport has a recognizable form which can be taught and learned, and it always has a defined aim or purpose. Participants may be individuals or teams, and the activity usually involves an element of competition. For instance, kick-about football in the street or local park might be classified as children's play, whereas matches between two teams played on a pitch under the direction of a referee are organized sport. Skateboarding and roller-skating, in themselves, can be considered physical activities or forms of exercise, but they are classified as sports when they are regulated into competition format.

Although we distinguish between sports and physical exercise activities done for their own sake, we consider both of relevance to children. Because we are taking sports to mean activities involving physical effort, we shall automatically be dealing with physical exercise as well, when we describe the concepts and problems relating to children's participation.

Why do children take up sports?

For the most part, children become involved in organized sports under the influence of adults. This is especially true when a child is very young, in the under-5 and under-10 age brackets, when there are practical constraints on the child's freedom of movement and therefore freedom of choice of activities. Even in the teenage years, children usually choose to do particular sports because of adult influences:

1. Children may take up sports which their parents or an influential adult have encouraged them to do.
2. A child's interest in a particular sport can be aroused by seeing the sport performed, perhaps in a local park or sports centre, or on television.
3. Physical education is an element in the school curriculum, so most children are introduced to organized sport compulsorily by their teachers when they start school at about the age of 5.
4. A sport may be chosen because there are convenient facilities for it, or because the parent or other adult is willing to take the child to the place.
5. Admiration for an adult who is good at a sport, whether a teacher, sports coach or star performer, can draw a child into that sport through a wish to identify with the attractiveness of performer or performance.
6. The lure of some sports' visible rewards, such as medals, trophies, fame, honours and money, can inspire children, especially older ones, to try to emulate top performers.

Adults may encourage children into sports for a wide variety of reasons. Governments often promote sports as a means of encouraging physical fitness which can then be channelled into a healthy army or an efficient workforce. Most countries have used fitness promotion programmes as part of more general health education programmes.[3–6] Some governments have promoted sporting excellence across a wide range of sports for the sake of national prestige.[7] As parent, coach or physical education teacher, you may perceive different sports as fostering a variety of qualities in children, including healthy growth, physical fitness, physical skills, tactical skills, survival skills, pride of performance, self-esteem, sportsmanship, teamwork, individuality, concentration, dedication, determination, competitiveness and aggression.

The reasons why adults might encourage children to do sports can be categorized broadly into four areas:

1. Sport for pleasure.
2. Sport for health benefits.

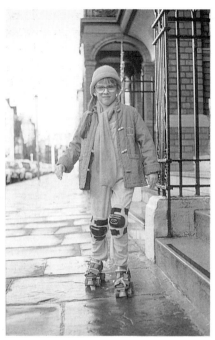

Roller-skating is fun – and good balance training.

3. Sport as specialized competition.
4. Sport for a possible future career.

One of these four categories may be the sole factor affecting the child's participation in sport, but there is often overlap between them. For instance, a child might be encouraged to take up athletics to help a medical problem like asthma, and then be motivated towards competing through discovering unexpected talent.

Sport brings children pleasure and entertainment through active participation. Children get bored very easily, especially when they are very young. Conversely, any activity which absorbs a child's attention provides entertainment. So, provided the sport is enjoyable and requires full participation (avoiding boring lulls), it will give the child pleasure. You may be involved in occupying children's time with sports as a teacher or a parent.

If you are a teacher, you often have a problem with numbers, and you may have to accept that not all the children in a group will be equally entertained by a particular sport. One of the skills of physical education teaching is successfully to involve all the children in a group in the game or sport, despite their varied abilities, characters and interests. You may have to organize different activities for different sections of a group. You have to choose sports or games which the children will enjoy and from which they will derive benefit.

As a parent, you have an easier task relatively, and children are readily drawn into sports encouraged within their families. Swimming is an example of a sporting activity which all members of a family can share, even when the youngest are still babies. You may want to encourage your children to take up sports which you enjoyed when you were small, or those sports which you wish you could have done, had you had the opportunity or facilities. Sport can be used as a family activity, or as a means of allowing a child independent entertainment.

Sport can promote physical fitness, good posture, good health and mental relaxation, through its component of physical exercise. The relationship between exercise and health benefits has been the subject of intense study, and, in the main, the conclusions have been that exercise does provide these benefits.[8-11] Young children, unlike adults, may not perceive an increased sense of well-being after active exercise, so they may not have a particular motivation to do sport as against spending hours watching television or videos, unless adults persuade them otherwise. As a physical education teacher, you may have to overcome resistance to the idea of physical exercise. Your choice of activities has to be attractive to pupils at different stages of

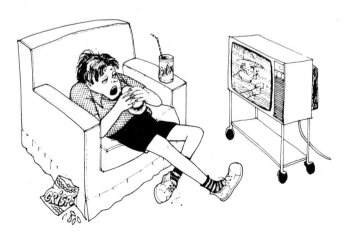

physical and emotional development. It is often easier to persuade teenagers to do sport or exercise on the grounds that it will make them look slimmer and more attractive, than to interest them in the traditional rivalries involved in competitive school team games.

In most countries, concern has been expressed about the effects of a sedentary lifestyle on the health of adults. The worry is not only that habitual inactivity and lack of exercise can lead to heart disease, but that it can also harm the body's bone structure.[12] The concern has spread to children, as evidence grows that children's lifestyles are increasingly inactive, and this may have long-term ill-effects on their health.[13] Increasingly, physical educationists and medical specialists are encouraging the use of sports and exercise for children to combat future ill-health, in the hope that the habit of exercise will last into adulthood. If you, as a parent, have taken up exercise for your own health benefit, you will probably involve your children as a matter of course.

Sport as specialized competition can bring a variety of rewards, whether physical, emotional or material. The example of successful performers is a powerful one in motivating children to take up a particular sport. There was a sudden surge of involvement in girls' gymnastics in Britain, following Olga Korbut's gold-medal-winning elfin performances in the 1972 Olympics. Parents may be impressed by the attractiveness of the sport and its performers. You may wish to see your child attaining similar levels of achievement and fame. This is part of your natural wish as a parent to 'obtain the best' for your child.

As a coach, you may be impressed by a child's talent, and you may be in the position of advising the parent on how the child can develop a competitive career to take advantage of that talent. You probably have to be careful to warn of the possibility of failure for the child, while encouraging both child and parents to aim at the top, if it seems attainable. You may wish to take control of the child's sporting activities, and therefore most of the child's free time, but you have to allow for the child's schooling, family relationships and other interests.

Sport as a career may be a good option for the young talented player, especially for the child who expresses little interest in other possible careers, or who has no particular academic bent. In many sports, life as a teaching professional offers a fair income, and recognized qualifications or certificates are readily available to suitable players who wish to pursue a career as professional sports coaches. There are various options for the paid professional, ranging from work in schools, sports centres or clubs, with individuals, or with teams or squads as the specialist governing body coach.

Parents or other influential adults may view sport as a good way for the child to make a larger than normal income. As the barriers between amateur and professional sports have broken down, helped by the International Olympic Committee's acceptance of 'open' sports such as tennis within the previously strictly amateur Games, the financial rewards for top performers in many sports are visibly on a par with the earnings of pop stars or other famous entertainers, and far in excess of normal wages in most forms of employment. Occasionally, sport provides an opening for a mediocre performer with a strong personality to become a media star: for instance, Eddie 'the Eagle' Edwards reportedly earned very large sums of money after coming last in the ski jump at the Calgary Winter Olympics in 1988.

As a parent, you may feel the potential financial rewards in sport are the determining factor in your choice of sports for your child. World squash champion Ross Norman used to remark in jest that he would encourage any talented future child of his own into tennis rather than squash, as it was easier to make a 'good' living as a professional tennis player. For some parents, the choice of sport for your child is a serious long-term calculation. The far-sighted adult is aware of the future pressures involving both athletic performance and financial arrangements, and plans both sides together.[14]

Why do we worry?

One aspect of concern in children's sport is whether children do the right kinds of sport or physical exercise, especially at school, and whether they get enough exercise in the context of modern lifestyles where physical convenience is a dominant factor. More worrying are the special problems attached to children participating in elite competitive sport before they have the physical or mental maturity to make independent judgements about their activities. As a parent, you have to be aware of the danger that your child might not join the small elite who achieve success and big earnings in sport. You also have to foresee that your relationship with your child might change with the years: there may be resentment later if you have channelled your child into one activity to the exclusion of others, however good your intentions. The coach faces similar dilemmas: you might deprive the child of invaluable and essential experiences if you have limited his or her activities to a single sport.

Because it is acknowledged that skills are most efficiently learned by the very young, early specialization in sport has long been the norm in most competitive sports in most countries. In some countries, notably East Germany (as it was until 1990) and the Soviet Union, talent spotting and selection of potential stars has been refined by technology: training analyses are done on computers to assess young competitors' progress, so that the best talents are discovered through a continual monitoring process.[15] Some countries have specialist sports schools: in Britain there is a football training centre for top juniors at the Lilleshall National Sports Centre, and an exclusive 'tennis school' for a very few selected promising young players at the Bisham Abbey National Sports Centre. India and Australia have National Institutes of Sport.[16, 17] One major problem of identifying youthful talent in order to nurture it in a special environment is the problem of failure: how does the child cope if he or she does not succeed, whether in competitions or within the inevitably increasingly harsh system of selection within the institution itself? Another problem is the isolation of the child from the normal groups of other children who would be friends or acquaintances in an ordinary school.

Top-level and even lower-level competitors tend to be isolated: the need for determination and concentration, combined with the constant travelling involved in most modern sports, make it difficult to sustain close relationships or friendships. Sixteen-year-old tennis star Monica Seles, interviewed after winning the German Open Championships in 1990, spoke of the antagonism most of her fellow-professionals seemed to show her. Footballer Diego Maradona apparently had to book the whole restaurant if he wanted to eat out in Naples without being disturbed by his fans when he was at the height of his fame in the late 1980s. Politics can add to the isolation: both Ivan Lendl and Martina Navratilova left their native Czechoslovakia to settle in the United States in order to pursue their tennis careers. When East European communism suddenly altered at the end of 1989, there were reports that top East German sports stars were coming under verbal and physical attack from people who resented their supposed wealth and privileges. Victims were said to include swimmers Kristin Otto and Heike Friedrich, cyclist Uwe

Ampler, discus thrower Martina Hellmann and speed skater Constanze Moser.

Parents and coaches often blame each other for a child's failures and disappointments in sport.[18, 19] Sometimes the child, once grown, can identify a different cause for de-motivation in a competitive sports career, blaming not individuals, but the administration and coaching policies of the sport's governing body. One formerly promising junior British tennis player condemned the Lawn Tennis Association (LTA), while recognizing her own early mistakes, in a letter to former tennis champion Angela Buxton, written when the player was 23: 'I was desperately unhappy with life on the circuit . . . I was so wrapped up in my world of training and practice that I neglected everything that was important to me, namely school and family. These two things, as I now realize, are vital for a 16-year-old . . . The problem was that everything was so easy and I think I took a lot for granted – the LTA paid for trips and arranged things for me . . . I think that where the system breaks down is when you reach 18 as it is then up to you and it really hits you hard. The LTA don't really want to know you as you are not a junior any more, but to me the first two years out of juniors are probably where you learn most of all and when you need all the help there is . . . I feel frustrated that I never reached my full potential – how many British players honestly do? . . . Can it be a coincidence that of all the girls I grew up with, only one is playing successful full-time tennis . . . and she happened to complete her schooling before starting her tennis career.'[20]

Anybody who influences a child's formative years can be a force for evil as well as good. As a parent, you have to take care whom you trust with your child's welfare, in case the child is subjected to sexual interference, whether heterosexual, homosexual or lesbian. Very young children might attract the paedophile, while teenagers, often unwittingly, might seem seductive to unscrupulous adults in close contact with them.

If as coach or parent you make mistakes in relation to a child's sport, these are rarely rectified at the time. You may think that warnings of harm from impartial observers are insulting your judgement. You can subject children to enormous pressure to succeed, often without realizing it. As coach, you have to be aware of the child's long-term interests, both within and outside sport, and at the same time you have to relate to the child's parents. Many coaches dealing with children in sports clubs or centres are unpaid volunteers:[21] if the relationship between child and coach or parent and coach breaks down, this can lead to bitterness and resentment.

Parents – oppressive or supportive?

While the influence of a coach can be great, it is magnified if you also happen to be the child's parent. Sometimes, parents' motivation is selfish, although this is generally unconscious. Parents might find reflected glory in their child's aspirations and successes in a high-profile sport.[22] This can be part of a situation in which the child is given the responsibility of achieving ambitions which the parents feel they missed out on in their own youth. The possibility of vast earning power can tempt parents or coaches to put a child under great pressure to excel in a particular sport because of its potentially high rewards, even if the child happens to prefer a different sport. Some adults may also unscrupulously ensure for themselves a share of the child's future earnings, before the child is capable of understanding the implications of contracts and business dealings.

Even on the simplest levels, your role as parent may not correspond happily with your role of provider, adviser, coach, supporter, and back-up team for your child's sports participation.[23, 24] The demands of a sport can be detrimental to normal family life. For instance, in Britain practice and training sessions for sports like gymnastics, ice-skating and swimming tend to take place very early in the morning, or late in the evening, because of pressure on facilities. Most sports competitions involve travelling, sometimes long distances, so parents or other adults are inevitably cast in transport and supervision roles, which are both expensive and time-consuming. Often, the whole of family life is dominated by the sporting ambitions of one or more of the children. Occasionally, parents allow this situation to develop inadvertently, and then it continues because they do not want to disappoint the child. If you concentrate on one child who is specially talented or keen, other children in the family may feel neglected. All too often, one or both parents have identified with the child's ambitions, and become totally engrossed in furthering them. If you become too involved with your child's sport, your child is likely to feel stifled and wish you had some activities of your own to divert your attention away. In some cases, parental ambition exceeds that of the child, leading to a situation in which the child continues the sport through filial duty alone, without deriving personal pleasure or pride from it.

The following real-life examples show how parents and children can relate in different ways, with very differing results, in the context of children's sport.

Greg. A desire to please his father motivated Greg to play serious competitive squash. His father played the game, and taught his sons. It was the only game Greg could beat his older brother at, and he felt it helped him to form a special bond with his father. Greg's brother was naturally talented for sports, and he played basketball for the national team. He resisted all the pressure put on him by his father to concentrate on serious sport, preferring to aim at an academic career. Greg, on the other hand, gave up football at the age of eleven to concentrate on squash.

Throughout his childhood, Greg felt that his father placed immense pressure on him to succeed at squash. Greg dreaded going home if he had lost a match, but even if he won, he was made to feel that he had not achieved enough for his father. Although he reached the top national junior ranks, he did not feel his squash career was a success.

Eventually, Greg left home, and came under the influence of the legendary Australian coach Len Steward. In the space of a year, Greg's squash improved greatly, but he did not have the financial resources to become a professional tournament player, so at the age of 19 he decided to drop out of squash, and spent three years driving trucks around Europe. He then started playing squash again, because he felt he wanted to play 'for himself'. But he found he was losing matches he ought to win, and felt his mental attitude was negative, allowing him to find excuses for losing instead of positive motivation. He consulted a sports psychologist, but to no avail, although he discovered that part of his problem was a subconscious lingering desire to play 'to prove things to his father'. He then tried hypnotherapy, which brought immediate results in boosting his confidence through positive self-awareness. His results improved, and he began to climb up the world rankings again.

Greg also enjoyed coaching squash, and he was appointed coach to a junior County squad, which consisted of about thirty-six of the region's best juniors. Representative teams were chosen from the squads, and the best players would have the chance to make national teams. Greg was horrified to find the intensity of pressure some parents applied to their squash-playing children. He saw his own experiences mirrored in theirs, and felt deep sympathy for the children. One father, who was totally involved with squash, and whose wife was a squash coach, telephoned Greg one day claiming that his relationship with his son was perfect, and that he was not pressurizing him to succeed in squash. The son telephoned Greg later, in tears because of the pressure he felt was being applied to him. He was 18. Another father was constantly boasting of the brilliant squash achievements of his 8-year-old son, and disagreed with Greg's feeling that a child of that age should be playing with toys and having fun, rather than trying to beat his father's contemporaries at squash. After three years, Greg found himself thoroughly depressed by these experiences. He tried to resign, but was persuaded to stay on. The following year, the parents' committee which controlled the County squad asked him to leave, because they resented his open disapproval of their interference.

Mike McIntyre and Bryn Vaile. When Mike McIntyre won the gold medal for Star Class yachting at the Seoul Olympics in 1988, at the age of 32, it was literally the culmination of a lifetime's ambition. His first reaction was to consider retiring from competitive sailing, but this was never a serious possibility. The following year, he was part of the winning Admiral's Cup team. He was left wondering what competitive goals were left: the only peak he could identify to aim at next was the America's Cup.

Mike had always been intensely competitive and ambitious. When he was 7, the family went to Kenya, and Mike and his two brothers learned to swim at a local club. Although the club offered coaching, Mike remembered teaching himself the back stroke, which became his best event. The three boys swam in competitions, and, to a certain extent, competed with each other. Their parents were keen for them to have every opportunity for sports. They took the boys to events and supported their efforts to excel, although they never put any pressure on them, or made them feel badly if they did not win.

Neither of Mike's parents swam, nor did they sail. Mike's father was involved in competitive motor rallying, but this was one sport he did not encourage his children to do. When the family returned to Scotland, they found the facilities for swimming limited to an outdoor pool. They lived by the sea, however; friends suggested they should join them sailing, and before long the children had their own Mirror dinghy. Mike was just 11. As the boys grew older, their father gradually sacrificed his own sporting interests in order to buy his sons boats for their sailing events. This was not his only expense: when his youngest son John became interested in riding, he was given his own pony to compete on.

Their father, a professor of veterinary medicine, also encouraged the boys to aim at successful careers. John went on to play good class rugby alongside running his own business, while Peter continued sailing although his appointment as a consultant gastroenterologist by the age of 35 left him little leisure time. Mike gained a first class honours degree in electronics and electrical engineering, but remained single-minded about his ambition to win Olympic gold. His decision to concentrate on sailing rather than swimming, begun through circumstances, was reinforced when he was 12 by the victory of Rodney Pattison and Iain Macdonald-Smith in the Flying Dutchman Class at the 1968 Olympics.

Mike's initial ambition was in the Finn Class, which he felt was the ultimate: 'one man and his machine against the rest'. However, he was disappointed with achieving only seventh place in the 1984 Games, having started as favourite, so he took the opportunity to transfer to the Star Class when, some ten months before the Seoul Olympics, crew-man Bryn Vaile offered him the chance to helm a competitive boat, loaned to Bryn by Swiss businessman Peter Erzberger.

Bryn and Mike were the same age, but contrasting and divergent characters, who knew each other only slightly before joining forces for their Olympic campaign. By coincidence, their early careers in sport showed similarities. Like Mike, Bryn was a successful County swimmer, and he enjoyed all competitive sports, especially cricket and rugby. As a child, Bryn was often isolated, through circumstances, so he loved the social aspects of sports as well. His adoptive parents were very keen on sport themselves, and they encouraged Bryn and his younger sister Terry. Golf was the only sport Bryn took a dislike to, giving up at the age of 12 because parental pressure to fulfil a serious training programme took the fun out of the game. Terry never took to golf, preferring tennis and riding, and she was bought her own pony at about the age of 12.

Bryn's father introduced the children to sailing, and Bryn was also able to sail at school. By the age of 11 he was showing special enthusiasm for the sport, and his father bought him a Mirror dinghy. Bryn's competitive swimming career peaked in the under-13 category, because a growth spurt when he was 12 made him relatively powerful; it ended when he found he was less successful in the under-15 competitions. The family went to Singapore for four years when Bryn was 15, and he was able to play a lot of rugby, squash and golf, which he found he now enjoyed. During his school summer holidays Bryn would return to Britain to take part in as many national sailing championships as possible, crewing in a variety of boats. Sailing became his dominant interest, encouraged by his father and others such as Club Commodore John Fisk.

Like Mike, Bryn was inspired by the 1968 Olympics, but his Olympic ambitions crystallized when he read Gary Hoyt's book *Go For Gold* at the age of 16. Also like Mike, Bryn tried the Finn Class, but could not achieve a satisfactory level of success as a helmsman. Both men learned a lot of sailing's technical aspects through experience, and were helped by having sailed in different types of boats. In contrast to Mike's search for a new challenge, Bryn continued his competitive career in the Star Class, aiming at further international and Olympic successes.

Mike felt that the route to the top would be easier for young British yachtsmen, who now had Youth Squads and technical and medical back-up teams, which were not available to Mike and Bryn in their early careers. Bryn, however, felt that squad coaching schemes could only help up to a point, whereas personal help and advice from people such as his own 'mentor' Vernon Stratton were invaluable for the development of a competitor's individual abilities.

In 1989, Bryn married Erika Lessmann, who continued her successful involvement with yachting after her marriage. Mike's wife Caroline, on the other hand, gave up sailing in 1980 after a spell crewing for her husband in a 505 – even though they won the series. After that, she continued to support Mike's efforts, and later devoted most of her time to looking after their two children, Angus and Gemma.

Both Mike and Caroline wanted their children to do a wide range of sports. They made jokes about buying Angus tennis rackets or golf clubs rather than a boat, because of the richer potential rewards in those sports. In fact, they were keen not to influence their children's choice of sports, except to the extent that they would not encourage them to do gymnastics, weightlifting or boxing, on the grounds that these carried risks of physical damage or the development of 'extreme body types'.

Mike and Caroline felt that parents should not be too closely involved in teaching their own children sporting skills, so they were very disappointed to find that no swimming lessons were available for under-5s at their local pool, due to excessive demand. During the year the family had spent in Australia while Mike was competing in the America's Cup event, Angus had almost learned to swim competently before he was 2. Mike and Caroline were also appalled at the lack of sports opportunities in British state schools, and this was an important factor when they decided on private education. They felt that there was too little sport in the state school programme, and it was not taken seriously enough.

Mike was glad that Angus showed a fiercely competitive spirit, even by the age of 4. He felt this was important, as one had to be competitive in all aspects of life, not just in sport, in order to do well relative to other people. Angus enjoyed football, cricket, rugby and golf (using little plastic clubs), but his great passion was sailing, following trips on the *Star* during the Olympic trials, and on *Juno* after the Admiral's Cup in 1989.

Mike was certainly willing to encourage Angus, and to help him in the same way as he had been helped by his own father. But he stated categorically that he would not be disappointed if his children were not especially successful in sport. Bryn and Erika were keen for their future children to have fun through sport alongside trying to achieve their own level of excellence. Mike and Bryn strongly agreed that their highest ambition for their children was for them to try their best in all their chosen activities, including sports.

The Page Family. When Cheryl Page was 11 years old, she hit the headlines of the national press in Britain through being refused entry to the London Marathon and several other official races, on the grounds that she was too young. The Amateur Athletic Association (AAA) operated an age limit of 18, and many medical specialists were called in to justify why marathon running was considered dangerous for children. The newspapers presented a sad story of a child being pushed into competitive marathon running by her father, a major in the British Army, because he wanted her to be an Olympic star and believed she needed an early start. The truth was rather different.

Cheryl was born in Hong Kong, and the family travelled widely when she was young. The family was close-knit, even though sister

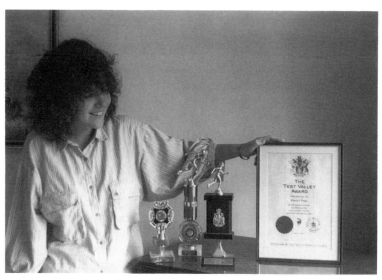

Cheryl Page with some of her awards.

Pamela was twelve years older than Cheryl. Parents Brian and Dorothy were not involved in competitive sport, although Dorothy had been proficient in folk-dancing contests in her native Scotland. Both Brian and Dorothy enjoyed being active, and swimming and walking were among the family's leisure pursuits.

While Pamela was more interested in music, Cheryl's obvious enthusiasm for sport was encouraged. She gained her bronze and silver Amateur Swimming Association awards, and many of the British Amateur Gymnastics Association standards. When the family was stationed in Germany for six years, there were ample opportunities for family sport. Walks at weekends were a feature of family life in Düsseldorf. Many walks in aid of selected charities were organized by the Church, for which Brian was chairman of the Mission Committee. Cheryl did her first at the age of 5, completing about 8 km as her mother would not allow her to do the whole 15 km. *Völkswandern* were walks organized by the German sports associations, with children encouraged by medals presented at the end of chosen distances. Cheryl loved the atmosphere of treasure hunt, combined with walks through the beautiful forests in the company of lots of new friends.

When the family was moved to Berlin, running replaced the

walking, partly because Brian needed training for his Army Fitness Test. Cheryl ran in her age-group events, covering $\frac{1}{2}$–1-mile distances, but she found these frustrating, because she would finish low in the field, but still fresh. Two boys in her class were running in the longer, grown-up events, and it was largely their boasting which inspired Cheryl's move into longer-distance running. At the age of 9, she ran her first 13-km race in fifty-five minutes. At 10, she did her first marathon, in Berlin, encouraged by the organizers, and she enjoyed the experience hugely.

The family's return to England when Cheryl was 11 brought a change to their sporting activities. There were no facilities locally for swimming or gymnastics. When Cheryl arrived at a local marathon event with her father, she was refused official entry, so she ran 'unofficially', without receiving a medal or crossing the finishing line. She was able to join in 'People's Marathons' officially, but these were not always convenient, so she joined in several more AAA events unofficially. Brian and Dorothy felt that if Cheryl wanted to run long distances, including marathons, she should be allowed to do so providing this did not interfere with her academic and general life progress, and that it was not in any way damaging her health.

She would usually run about three marathons a year, and her training never amounted to more than about 30–40 miles per week. By the age of 13, her best marathon time was three hours thirty-seven minutes, and by 15 she had completed fourteen marathons. Trying to encourage Cheryl's enthusiasm and to channel it properly, the family sought the guidance of an official athletics coach, but Cheryl did not survive an interview in which the coach insisted that he must have total control of her running, and that she abandon long distances to run in mile events, despite her insistence that she did not enjoy the shorter distances in which she did not excel. Cheryl decided that this approach was not for her.

Looking back, at the age of 18, Cheryl had fond memories of the fun she had had doing walking and running events, especially in Germany. All her marathons were run for different charities, and she felt that this gave her a sense of purpose. Dorothy and Brian were proud that Cheryl had earned some £11,000 for worthy causes through her running, gaining in the process the 1986 National Child of Achievement Award and the 1988 Test Valley (Hampshire) Community Award. Neither Cheryl nor her parents had ever approached running with serious ambitions for later success, although in her own words Cheryl was, even at 11, a 'determined, complete perfectionist'. The family was still perplexed by the strong opposition Cheryl's running interests had aroused, and equally disappointed by the lack of sporting opportunities they had found in Britain.

In fact, Cheryl's chief aim had always been to become an actress, and she won many national awards for speech and drama, besides prizes for essay-writing. Her father dissuaded her from Stage School, insisting that she should get an academic degree first and then take up acting if she still wished, to keep her career options open. At 15, Cheryl suddenly developed a debilitating viral infection, shared by a few other girls at her school, and possibly linked to a contaminating spillage in the local water supply. From having never been ill or injured before, Cheryl found that she was too tired to do more than survive each day, never mind run. After three years, she was just beginning to recover. However, she still gained excellent examination results to earn her university place, and was aiming at a career as a barrister.

Cheryl's running was also reviving after the illness. She still felt too weak to run in the mornings, when her father normally did his running, but she had started to run two or three times a week with a friend, and they did a half-marathon together in aid of charity. She was looking forward to feeling fit, sharp-minded and clear-headed again, as she had felt through her childhood running.

The Carter Family. Cyril Carter is a sportswriter and teacher qualified in sports science, physical education, psychology and philosophy. He was formerly personal coach to two of Britain's star judo players, track and field coach at the University of Idaho in the United States, and national coach to the British Amateur Rowing Association. With coaching qualifications in nine different sports, he trained several top sportsmen in the different disciplines required for the television 'Superstars' competitions.

As a parent and educationist, Cyril decided that he wanted his daughter Sharon to do sport, within the broader aim of providing for her physical, intellectual, social and spiritual development. His ultimate aim for Sharon, and subsequently for her little sister Christina, was to 'maximize their potential for choice, success and happiness', while developing them into 'kind, sympathetic and happy human beings'.

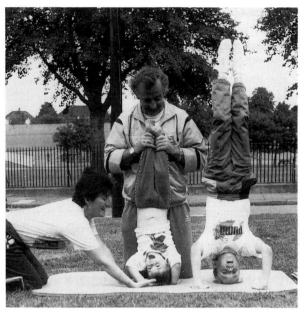

The Carter family.

Cyril's aim was for Sharon to be competent in a range of sporting skills, so that she could enjoy sports, and socialize through them. He also admitted freely that he would love her to win an Olympic gold medal for athletics, or better still the Wimbledon tennis tournament. He felt that tennis offered the greatest scope for good players to earn good money, and it had the added advantage of being a very sociable game which could be played throughout life.

He formulated his aim into a thoroughly prepared 'programme for life', based on his own knowledge and experience of sports participation and coaching. The core of the programme was to combine swimming, gymnastics and athletics, starting at the age of 3. Details were calculated: a year could contain a potential maximum of 224 swimming sessions, 160 periods of gymnastics and 96 stints of athletics. Other sports would be added to the programme later.

Cyril's wife Rita, also a teacher, had never done any sport herself, but she learned to swim with her baby daughter. Rita agreed with Cyril's idea of setting out a long-term programme, but felt that Sharon should join sports clubs, instead of doing everything under her parents' guidance. In Cyril's words, Rita became his best critic, and she agreed with every step he took.

Having tried three gymnastics clubs in five years, Cyril was adamant that Sharon should learn gymnastics, one of his own sports, without the pressure of attending a club which would inevitably mean intensive training and competitions. Sharon also joined a swimming club, which she thoroughly enjoyed, and gained 'Silver Squad' standard and age-group County qualifying times by the age of 10. However, the club penalized her by demoting her squad rating because she could not attend all the training and competition sessions. Therefore her parents withdrew her, on the grounds that the club was trying to force her to specialize, over-train and over-compete at the expense of her education and need for sleep.

By the time she was 10, Sharon had gained over 500 personal performance awards in many sports, including canoeing, trampolining and life-saving, with six Five-Star Amateur Athletic Association awards. She was the youngest achiever of several awards: at the age of 6 she earned the Royal Life Saving Society's Aquagold Award, and at 7 the Amateur Swimming Association (ASA) Ultimate Swimmer Award, the International Swimming Teachers' Diploma, and the ASA's distance award for completing 10,000 metres.

Sharon was also a competent gymnast, and she enjoyed horse-riding regularly. She had tried a little short tennis, and was just beginning golf. She was not allowed to neglect her school-work, either, and her parents were considering whether she should apply for a scholarship to a good secondary school, such as Millfield, where she could pursue her sports and gain a sound academic education.

The cost of the family's sport was a heavy burden, especially when second daughter Christina was added to the 'programme for life', starting swimming at $3\frac{1}{2}$ months. Sponsorship was found, which provided sports clothing and equipment, and a certain amount of financial help, although not enough to pay for extras such as physiological monitoring.

There was also television and press publicity, which gave rise to some criticism of Cyril's methods from medical specialists and sports coaches. Cliff Temple, athletics coach and journalist, condemned a sponsor's press release offering 'demonstrations of Sharon's prowess' when she was 6, and concluded one of several critical articles with the statement that there would be no press release about his playing football in the back garden with his own 7-year-old! (*Running* magazine, no. 74, June '87.) In fact, Cyril himself was not happy about the press release, but it was distributed without his knowledge.

Cyril Carter asked himself fundamental questions such as 'what is important to the healthy development of modern-day children?' and 'what can I, as a parent, offer my child?' Within the physical side of his 'programme for life', his aims were to give his daughters a broadly-based grounding in several, different sports; to teach them the specific skills of those sports; to underpin this with good body conditioning, with suppling as the priority; and to leave them with open options as to whether they wished to continue sport purely for pleasure or to pursue top-level competitive careers, should they be good enough, when they grew up.

The broader aim of this multi-sport, skills-based approach was to bridge the normally accepted dichotomy between sports and physical education. If successful, the experiment might develop and come to be accepted by sports coaches and physical education teachers as the safe alternative to pushing children towards hopes of sporting success through early specialization, over-intensive training and excessive age-group competition. The method could still allow successful competitive specialization, but at a much later stage than was currently the vogue in British sport.

2 Body Conditioning and Fitness Training

Selection of games and sports

Sports and games provide children with healthy physical exercise, and therefore help them to be physically fit. But there is a limit to the amount of fitness any one sport can provide, as some sports require and develop strength, others flexibility, others eye–hand co-ordination. Many sports entail a combination of several fitness parameters. If the child is encouraged to do sports in order to be or get fit, several sports should be chosen, in order to provide the different aspects of physical well-being, and to avoid the injury risks inherent in doing just one type of exercise. Selecting various types of physical activity for your child is a process which can begin at the earliest age. Opportunity is one major factor in the child's development of physical skills. Imitation is another, and it is often the case that younger children learn skills at an earlier age than the first-born because they copy from the older child. Some children are fearless, and will happily clamber over ropes and climbing frames by the age of 18 months, whereas others may be more circumspect, gradually gaining confidence as they experience new movements. Some never overcome nervousness of heights or fears of falling. A child may show special talent for certain skills, such as catching or hitting a ball, while another may always miss: in either case, the child should still be encouraged to enjoy playing with a ball, without special pride or inhibition.

You can teach your baby to paddle and swim in a warm pool as early as 3 months old, after the major vaccinations have been done. The baby can learn to swim comfortably under water, but may then find it harder to learn the co-ordination involved in swimming and breathing on the surface. Once a baby is walking, he or she becomes very active naturally, and will take any opportunity offered to run, or

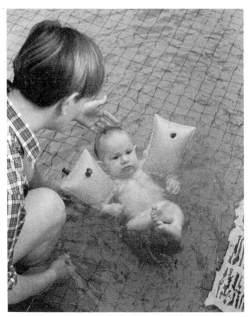

'Swimming' lessons can start from the earliest age.

to kick or hit a ball. Throwing and catching a ball are skills which develop slightly later. Riding a push-tricycle is an early-stage activity, but the child might learn to turn the pedals on a tricycle or a bicycle with stabilizers from the age of about 18 months. By the age of 4 or 5, the child might be able to balance and ride a bicycle. 'Tumble-tot' gymnastics is a modern teaching system designed to introduce very young children to basic gymnastic exercises and manoeuvres. Children who live in snowy climates have usually learned to ski by the age of about 3.

A range of basic skills gives the child a chance to try a wide variety of formal sports later on, even in the absence of special talents. The question of when a child might be introduced to competitive sport, and whether the child should specialize if he or she seems talented for a competitive sport, is difficult to solve. This author believes that team and individual competitions for young children, up to the age of about 12, or even up to 16, should be strictly for fun, and played on a round-robin rather than knock-out basis: for instance, every entrant in a short tennis tournament should receive a prize, regardless of who might be the overall winner. If you encourage your child into a

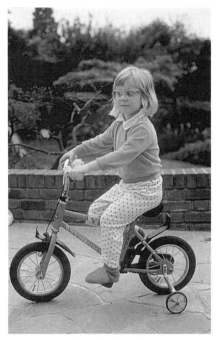

Learning to cycle.

sport as a potential future career, you must be sure that you have really weighed up carefully whether the child will be capable of a career in professional sport, and will be able to cope with the stresses involved. A key question must be: how will the child manage if he or she is injured or ill and cannot play?

As later chapters will make clear, over-specialization is dangerous for body development, laying aside any possible emotional or psychological problems. If a child wants to specialize in a sport, he or she must get fit for that sport, like any adult, partly in order to perform better within the necessary parameters, and partly to avoid the injury risks involved in doing a particular type of movement or through repeated body stresses. The specialist sport itself should not be used for fitness training. This is equally true if the sport involves repetitive stress, like running, swimming or rowing, or varied stresses as in tennis, football, hockey or throwing events, where rotational movements can cause spinal distortion. For the younger child, fitness training is simply incorporated in different exercise activities.

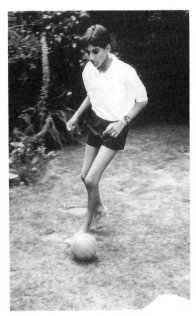

Practising football skills.

The teenager should be told the reasons for doing certain types of fitness training, and their relevance to the main sport. The background to sports specialization can be either sports or formal fitness training. At any age, combinations of other sports as in the triathlon, pentathlon and decathlon groupings carry less risk of injury than sports pursued singly, such as running, swimming or tennis. The advantage of formal training is that it can be strictly controlled, and can include specific protective exercises.

Posture

This is the body's basis for activity, and all human posture is achieved against the effect of gravity. The body's muscles have to support the weight of the limbs and trunk against the load of gravity. When they activate to create movements, they work either *concentrically*, shortening against gravity, or *eccentrically*, lengthening out to control the movement against gravity's influence. When a child stands evenly on two feet, with the feet slightly apart, the loading is dissipated evenly down the central line of the body, whereas the loading is concentrated to one side if the body weight is shifted more over one leg. The body's postural, fatigue-resistant muscles are constantly active while the body is upright, whether sitting or standing. However, like other muscles, they are trained by usage. If the child develops bad postural habits, such as slouching, the postural muscles lose their proper tone, so it becomes progressively more tiring for the child to try to sit or stand straight with the head up. In both the short and the longer term, this has a bad effect on the body's joints, which can become distorted because they are not properly supported by the postural muscles.

Sport and exercises have a good training effect on the muscles they involve, but good posture has to be cultivated separately, as it requires a different type of muscle work. Many sports can create unsatisfactory postural habits: rowers and cyclists tend to have rounded shoulders, for instance. Throwing and racket sports create one-sidedness which results in an in-built twist in the spine. Some sports, such as gymnastics and diving, engender a more satisfactory erect posture. From the earliest age, a child should be encouraged to sit and stand straight and symmetrically, with head up, shoulders level and back, trunk erect and hips and knees level. Conversely, children should never be allowed to slouch or sprawl when sitting still, whether for meals or while reading or watching television. Chairs, tables and desks at school or at home should be adjusted to the correct height to encourage the child to sit properly upright at every stage of growth. This is specially important for the teenager studying for examinations.

There is no absolute criterion for good posture, and in fact it varies considerably according to the child's individual build, but its opposite, bad posture, is easy to recognize and should always be corrected.

Fitness training

This consists of several parts. A fitness programme should be tailored to the individual child, and planned as a progressive, finite schedule. It should be adaptable, in case the child finds it boring or difficult to achieve. It has to allow for rest, relaxation and recovery from effort. A training schedule might be set for a specific purpose like reducing weight in an obese child, or improving fitness in a child who does no sport, or who is a sports competitor. It is possible to introduce even young children to training, but formal training is most appropriate to older teenagers who know they need to get fitter for health purposes or sport. Any parent or coach setting a fitness programme for a child should obtain advice from a sports physiologist or physiotherapist. Monitoring the child's progress through physiological and biomechanical tests is vital. Examples of these types of tests are given in later chapters. If the child seems to retrogress, the programme must be modified or curtailed. Piling on more work when the child is over-tired can push him or her into injury or illness.

Aerobic fitness training is usually achieved by exercising fairly energetically for a period of twenty to thirty minutes. Running, cycling, skipping and swimming are suitable, but you have to remember the dangers of repetitive training, especially for teenagers, who are vulnerable to bone injuries (p. 116). The child has to build up gradually to twenty or thirty minutes, starting with only one session a week and increasing to three sessions, if required. It is unwise for a child to do more than three weekly sessions of the same activity, but a combination of running, cycling and swimming done alternately can provide aerobic fitness training on a daily basis.

Circuit training. A circuit is a series of exercises done at speed, with a short recovery between each exercise. It is an efficient training

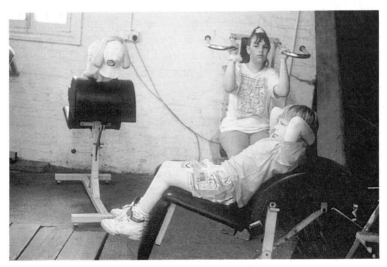

Children circuit-training on the Norsk equipment.

method for improving both aerobic fitness and muscle endurance. If the exercises are carefully chosen, body balance is considered, and protective movements can be included. Circuit training can also be done on gym equipment such as the Norwegian Norsk system. A circuit can be organized as exercises done a specific number of times, for instance fifteen or twenty repetitions, or done in a time, such as twenty or thirty seconds. The 'rest' period between each exercise, during which the child keeps moving about, or walks or runs to the next exercise station, should be about ten seconds, and the overall time spent on the circuit should be thirty minutes, although the child may build up to this from a starting point of five minutes. Interval training is done on a similar basis to this kind of circuit training, but the rest interval is usually equal to the exercise time span: for instance, the child may do thirty seconds of each, building up from six to twelve work–rest exercise bursts, and then increase the work–rest time to forty seconds, then forty-five seconds, each time starting with six intervals and gradually building up to twelve.

Speed and power work. Speed training comprises very short bursts of high-intensity activity, such as a ten-second sprint, with a relatively long recovery, perhaps fifty seconds, with the aim of avoiding the lactic acid incurred in anaerobic training (p. 44). Speed work can be done for the arms or legs, or both, and the child builds up gradually from about ten bursts of explosive work in a speed session. Power is a combination of speed and strength, so a child involved in sports like karate, sprinting, jumping or throwing events may need to do both types of training in order to improve. Strength training involves overloading muscles in order to increase their capacity. It can be done through overload exercises, such as running with weights round the wrists and ankles, or practising golf swings or tennis strokes with an abnormally heavy club or racket. The hydraulically resisted 'swim-bench' is another type of overload directly related to a sport. However, in adults and children alike one has to be careful not to overload the spine excessively as it rotates or twists, so there is a strict limit to the amount of weight-resistance one can use for this type of movement. It is safer to do progressive resistance training using 'straight-line' weight training, hydraulic resistance equipment, or body-loaded exercises such as press-ups or pull-ups to a bar.

Weight training. Modern weight training equipment like the Nautilus, David, Schnell and Norsk systems has made resistance training safer, as the body movements are well defined, and the starting positions are fixed, with the body and (usually) the head held in a correct, supported position. Most modern systems encourage a full range of movement, starting from a stretched position, which reduces the risk of muscle-bound tightness developing. The Norsk Sequence-Training system has the added advantage that the system is designed to cultivate a good and symmetrical balance of muscles throughout the body. Hydraulic resistance systems like Hydrafitness are excellent for concentric muscle endurance work, and largely avoid the risk that a child might be tempted to work beyond his or her capacity, although the lack of eccentric muscle work has to be compensated for with other exercises. Even using free weights, children can safely start weight or resistance training at a very early age – provided that they learn the techniques correctly, never handle a load they have to struggle to move, and that they are always supervised in the gym. Heavy resistance training, on the other hand, is not suitable for children during their growing periods, and so should not be recommended before the age of about 18. For the sports of weightlifting and powerlifting, this author believes that even young children can safely learn the techniques of the lifts, but they should not be allowed to lift to their maximum capacity in training or competition until they are fully grown.

Flexibility and mobility training. Sports like gymnastics and diving develop and require flexibility and mobility. Mobilizing exercises lubricate and loosen the joints and their soft tissues, and are usually done as rhythmical, bouncing movements. In the young child, mobilizing exercises also loosen the muscles. However, in the teenager, the muscles begin to tighten, and the only effective way to loosen them safely is through passive stretching exercises: the muscles are held absolutely still at their full length for a time (between five and thirty seconds); the stretch is then relaxed completely and repeated several times. The positions given as flexibility tests (exercises 5, 8, 11, 16, 17, 24, 26, 27, (pp. 101–13) can also be used as passive stretching exercises. Passive stretching routines are now considered vital for injury prevention, but not at the expense of muscle strength. Stength and flexibility have to be evenly balanced for effective body protection against stress and injury.

The warm-up. A warm-up is not really necessary for the very young child who is naturally active and plays games, but it is essential for sports like competitive gymnastics which involve intensive body workouts. Therefore the young gymnast is introduced to the discipline of warming up from the start. For many sports, the warm-up only becomes essential when the child is participating at a more serious level, and perhaps when the body changes following the growth spurt are evident. The warm-up consists of stretching, mobilizing and dynamic exercises, and possibly skill rehearsal for the older teenager in competitive sports. It has to last at least five minutes, and up to thirty minutes or longer if the environment is cold. The stretching element has to come first, if any muscles are particularly tight, or are recovering from injury; otherwise the warm-up can start with a jog or some dynamic exercises before the stretching. A warm-down on similar lines is useful for injury prevention after any hard exercise session.

Planning the programme. When a fitness programme is compiled for a child or teenager, its exact composition depends on the reasons for doing it. If the child has weaknesses such as inflexibility, priority is given to stretching and mobilizing exercises. If the child is training for a particular sport, the emphasis is on the fitness aspects that relate directly to the sport. Training should not interfere with skills practice or match play, so, if possible, the training schedule is designed to take place in the 'closed season' for the sport. On a daily basis, the activities are balanced: if the older teenager is training and playing intensively, for instance, hard sessions are followed by rest or gentler workouts. If different types of training are done on the same day, skills practice and speed training are done before circuit or weight training. The fitness schedule has to allow for rest and recovery, which means at least one day off intensive sports practice every week, and some longer rest periods at intervals during each year.

Protective exercises. These are designed to provide the body's muscles and joints with the correct balance of stability, mobility, strength and flexibility. A total protective exercise programme provides good body conditioning and helps good posture. It aims to balance the body, so that the legs or stomach are not relatively strong while the arms or back extensor muscles are weak, nor is one side of the body over-developed compared with the other side, nor is one muscle group tight or strong relative to its co-ordinating muscle groups. Protective exercises are worked out for the individual, and in relation to the individual's sport and its stresses, where relevant. The exercises described for biomechanical monitoring (p. 100) are among those suitable, and the child does more of those which he or she found most difficult, leaving out those which were very easy in the tests. When a child has had an injury, the protective exercises include remedial exercises specific to the injury. Following injury, or where particular weaknesses have been found through the biomechanical tests, the child should be encouraged to do the prescribed routine of protective and remedial exercises on a daily basis.

3 The Exercise Physiology of Children

By Craig Sharp

In most non-Third World countries there is concern regarding the physical fitness levels of school-age children. Indeed, in 1988, the School Sport Forum, a special committee sponsored by the British government, published its report *Sport and Young People: Partnership and Action*, in which it made wide-ranging recommendations aimed at increasing and improving children's participation in sport at all levels, from elite competition to basic health-promoting exercise.[1] The Forum was specially concerned to correct the drop-out rate from sport when children left school and no longer had easy access to sports facilities. Similarly, in the same year, the American College of Sports Medicine stated their opinion that physical fitness programmes for children and youth should be developed 'with the primary goal of encouraging the adoption of appropriate lifelong exercise behaviour'.[2] Thus there is a widespread impetus to engage children in sport and exercise, which is wholly commendable.

However, exercise extends into sport, sport extends into competition, and competition extends into elite performance, where children from 8 years old (or even younger) may be subjected to very strenuous exercise programmes. For example, a 7-year-old completed a full marathon race in three and a half hours, while a 13-year-old in the same race ran two hours fifty-five minutes.[3] Many other sports can involve children in intensive performance, including swimming, gymnastics, dance, track running, squash, rugby and football. Given that children can produce very high-level performances, and undergo the strenuous training required, it is important to consider some aspects of their exercise physiology.

Exercise physiology is the study of a whole variety of physical responses to exercise involving, for example, the heart, lungs, blood, muscle and metabolism. This is done by tests on people (technically termed 'subjects') using treadmills and cycle, canoeing, rowing, skiing and other ergometers (work machines). The subjects work as hard as possible while measurements are made of heart rate, oxygen consumption, carbon dioxide production and blood lactic acid, among other values. Through these tests, the exercise physiologist assesses the subject's fitness, and can advise on improving it. Fitness consists of several factors, including aerobic capacity (heart, blood and lungs), local muscle endurance (anaerobic capacity), muscle speed and strength, joint flexibility, and body composition in terms of percentage fat.

Children differ from adults in many of their body responses to hard physical activity, in that they are not just 'little adults' physiologically. In this chapter I shall describe important areas of difference relating to general body growth, body fat, muscle strength, muscle endurance, aerobic fitness, movement economy, flexibility and mobility, muscle versatility, heat control, dehydration and the child's view of exercise.

The skeleton and general growth

Before the adolescent growth spurt, boys and girls are much the same in their bone development, but between the ages of 10 and 13 years, girls develop more quickly than boys. They grow taller, heavier, and the trunk, in particular, increases in breadth and height. Following the trunk, the arms and legs grow longer, although they do not fill out until later. The hands and feet remain relatively slender compared to the growth of the trunk. From the age of 13, girls slow down as regards height development, whereas boys begin their pubertal growth spurt. After the age of 14, girls' annual growth rate slows down: they may even be fully developed with their adult characteristics by 14. Boys continue to grow rapidly until about 16 years of age, when their growth slows down.[4]

The long bones grow from the epiphyseal plates of cartilage near each end (p. 116). As a child grows, the body changes in its proportions. For instance, the foot is roughly half of its eventual full length when the child is about 18 months old, the vertebral column (backbone) reaches half its eventual height at about 2 years, and the leg attains half its full length roughly between 3 and 4 years.[5]

Different bones grow at different rates, and major developments happen in different areas of each bone. It has been recorded that in the arm, 80 per cent of the growth of the humerus (upper arm-bone) occurs at the proximal (upper) part of the bone, near the shoulder.[6] In the forearm, 75 per cent of the bone growth happens at the distal (lower) end of the radius (the bone on the thumb side), near the wrist. This means that less than 25 per cent of the growth of two of the three long arm-bones happens in the elbow region. In the leg, the growth pattern is virtually the reverse of the arm. In the femur (thigh-bone), 70 per cent of the growth happens at the distal end, near the knee, while 60 per cent of the tibia (shin-bone) growth and 55 per cent of the fibula (outer leg-bone) development happens at the upper end of the bones, again near the knee.

After the growth spurt, girls end up with a broader pelvis and hips, with the trunk proportionately longer in terms of sitting height, and relatively shorter legs compared with boys. The broader pelvis is one of the reasons why older girls throw out their heels when they run, as their thigh-bones have to create a greater angle to bring their knees close together. Boys end up with broader shoulders and longer arms at the end of their growth spurt. On average, 9-year-old boys are 3.5 mm broader across the shoulders (bi-acromial breadth) than girls, but by the age of 19 they are 37.3 mm broader.[4] Even quite small differences in shoulder breadth produce relatively large differences in upper trunk muscle mass, on the chest and upper back. This is partly why the strength differences between young adult males and females are much greater in the upper body than in the lower. The combination of stronger upper body muscle mass with the greater lever power of a longer arm gives boys an ultimate advantage in events such as the throws, canoeing, rowing, and racket sports.

The broadening of the shoulders in boys, and of the hips in girls, tends to raise the centre of gravity in the former, and to lower it in the latter. This gives girls greater stability and is one of the reasons why, in general, women have better balance than men, as exemplified by the balance-beam being a discipline of women's gymnastics, but not men's. Before puberty, children generally produce better performances than adults on tests of balance, such as the electronic stabilometer.

The growth areas of a child's bones can be badly disrupted by injuries. They can also be altered or harmed by excessive sports training. For instance, whereas a pronounced 'carrying angle' at the elbow may interfere with fluent motion for tennis serving or throwing events, there is some evidence that girls who do these sports seriously before puberty fail to develop the normal valgus angle, developing instead an abnormally straight arm, although the non-dominant arm bends outwards normally. On a much more serious level, various doping agents within the category of anabolic steroids may also cause damage by promoting premature calcification of the growth plates, if children take them before the epiphyseal plates have completed their growth. This can result in distortion or stunting of the child's bone growth. Anyone tempted to promote the use of anabolic drugs among young sports competitors, in defiance of their ban in most recognized sports, should bear in mind that the fusion process may not be finally over in all the bones until the age of about 25. Possible damage to growing bones is only one of many known harmful effects which might result from the use of these outlawed drugs.[7, 8]

While excessive sport, especially of a repetitive nature, might damage children's growing bones, it is known that even short periods of vigorous physical activity have beneficial effects on bone development in older children.[9]

Size, the growth spurt and puberty

From birth, children do not grow at an even rate. It is generally accepted that children's growth and development are less affected by poor exercise participation than by poor diet.[10] Interestingly, a study from Brazil comparing under-nourished and properly nourished boys from two districts of Rio de Janeiro showed that, although the mal-nourished boys were shorter and lighter, they performed better in tests of grip strength and vertical jump, but the better fed boys were superior in endurance tests.[11] This indicates how complex the study of children's physical capacities can be. Despite the evidence of this study, it would not be sensible to conclude that malnutrition is a positive aid to performance for junior high jump or strength events!

The growth spurt occurs approximately two years earlier in girls than in boys, commonly beginning between the ages of 10 and 12 years in the former, and 12 and 14 years in the latter, and stretching over about two years in each case. Thus, there is a stage when many girls will be bigger, heavier and possibly stronger than many boys of the same age. Girls may win events in mixed competitions where they would not be able to hold their own against males in older age groups. For instance, in a full-distance marathon race with age categories, girls won the 11- and 12-year age-groups, the latter in three hours, thirteen minutes and twelve seconds.[3]

Children of the same age and sex may be at very different stages in their growth, given that the growth spurt can start at any time over the two-year period. This reflects the difference between chronological age and biological age. One way of determining biological age fairly accurately is through X-rays of the vertebral column or the wrist, to show the degree of bone development (ossification)[12]. The relative mis-match of chronological and biological ages has important implications for age-group sport. Apart from the unfairness and possible physical dangers of matching children of similar ages but different development in sports like rugby and American football, some younger-maturing competitors, enjoying a relatively easy degree of early success, may become demoralized when their harder-training but slower-growing peers eventually catch up, while some later-maturing youngsters may give up sport altogether through discouragement at their early failures. This is where the more enlightened physical educationist or coach may have a major effect on a youngster's long-term future in exercise and sport.

In terms of bodyweight, it has been recorded that girls may gain an average total of 33.5 kg overall between the seventh and eighteenth years, while boys increase by 43.8 kg over the same period.[4] Bodyweight increases occur at different times in girls and boys: both sexes increase similarly between 7 and 10 years, with girls slightly lighter than boys. At about the age of 11, however, girls go ahead, gaining about 2 kg more than boys between the ages of 12 and 13. By the end of their fourteenth year, the boys have caught up.

In boys, the growth spurt usually coincides with the onset of puberty. At puberty, the boy's penis and testicles enlarge; hair grows in the pubic region, under the arms and on the face; the hair line on the temple recedes a little; the voice breaks and deepens, reflecting increased muscularity of the larynx; and the body muscles develop and enlarge. In girls, however, puberty usually comes only after the growth spurt is almost complete. At puberty, girls notice the growth of hair in the pubic region and under the arms; their body shape changes, with the development of the breasts and widening of the pelvis; and they start having periods.

Puberty in girls may be delayed by long spells of strenuous

physical activity in the pre-pubescent phase. It has been found that in competitive swimmers the onset of periods (menarche) was delayed by six months for every year of serious training before menarche: swimmers who started intensive training after menarche had begun to menstruate at 12 years 6 months, whereas those who had started training before menarche were 15 years old, on average, before they had periods. Among runners, girls who were training before menarche were, on average, 15 years 2 months when they had their first periods, while those who started training after menarche began to have periods at 12 years 9 months.[13] A delay in menarche involves a delay not only in menstruation but also in the growth of pubic and axillary hair, although mammary development may not be held up to the same extent. The pubescent, elfin-like appearance of some 15- or 16-year-old gymnasts usually owes much more to this form of natural delay due to intensive physical training than to puberty-delaying drugs, as has sometimes been suggested.

Physiologically, such a delay in menarche should not in itself be harmful, so the girls can usually expect a normal adulthood, with a normal chance of conceiving and giving birth to healthy children. However, if the young competitor has a delayed puberty together with amenorrhoea (total absence of periods), medical and nutritional advice should be sought.

Fat

Fat represents energy stored in fat cells in depots of *adipose tissue*. These are located under the skin (subcutaneously) in general, but particularly at specific sites such as the back of the arms, hips, thighs, abdomen and bust. Fat is estimated in various ways, including simple skinfold measures using callipers, and consists of from 5 to 40 per cent of a person's bodyweight. Chemical fats are present in blood, either as *free fatty acids*, which are fuel fats on their way to muscle, or linked to cholesterol.

During earlier childhood, girls have only slightly more body fat than boys.[14] For example, at the age of 8 a girl may have 18 per cent and a boy 16 per cent body fat. During and following the growth spurt, girls tend to put on fat, increasing it to about 25 per cent at 17, while boys tend to lose it, declining to 12–14 per cent at the same age. Some fat is essential as an energy source, to hold body organs in place, and to insulate nerves, among other functions. There is a very wide variation in body fat levels, not only between the sexes, but also

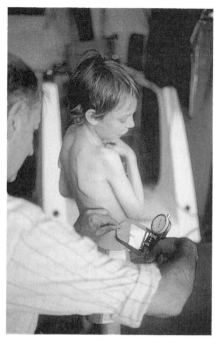

Skinfold measurement.

between individuals of the same sex. Young children are probably as fat as they look, but older children and adults who look slim may have surprisingly high percentages of body fat, and vice versa. A larger muscle covered by a little fat may look the same in size as a smaller muscle covered by a lot of fat. Also, it is not uncommon for older children to be both relatively fat and very fit, whereas slim children with low body fat are not necessarily as fit as they might appear.

Obesity can be defined as a much higher body fat percentage (in the order of 30 per cent or more) than that considered normal for the age and sex of the child. It may seem strange, but fat children are often not greedy in terms of overeating. Indeed, overweight adolescent girls may even have a lower calorie intake than others of so-called normal weight.[15] Lack of exercise is a vitally important factor: even in 6-month-old infants, percentage fat is positively related to lack of activity rather than to calorie intake.[16] In adolescence, lack of exercise or physical activity is a major cause of obesity. An increase in body fat occurs due to increases in fat cell size, or an increase in the number of fat cells, or both. Fat cells appear to increase in number until early adolescence, after which increases in body fat occur mainly by increasing the size of the existing adipose cells.

It may be possible to affect the development of fat cells during a child's growth by means of dietary manipulation, such as cutting down on sweets and 'junk food', together with an increase in exercise and physical activity such as walking. Fat children occur in both sexes, and 80 per cent of them go on to become fat adults. As indicated, fat children tend to take less exercise than their thinner counterparts, but, curiously, they also exercise less even when they are active. Obese children are handicapped by their excess weight, so they require a higher oxygen uptake to do a given task, yet their maximum oxygen uptake is often lower than that of leaner children.[17] Thus their available energy should be higher, but may be less than that of leaner children, which can give the impression that the obese child is not trying in the more active sports.

Children in general possess more of the heat-producing tissue known as 'brown fat', which is located under the skin, especially over the back. Brown fat, which diminishes as children get older, *may* have a weight-regulating function, acting as what might be termed a 'ponderostat'. It may control weight gain by diverting excess calories into heat rather than fat, for instance if the child overeats. It is possible that at least some obese children are born with relatively low brown fat levels.

While obesity is a problem related to lack of sufficient exercise, anorexia nervosa, or an obsession with excessive thinness, can be a problem directly linked to over-exercising.[18] It occurs mainly in female adolescents, although it can also affect boys. In many sports, relatively low body fat is obviously desirable, but this should not be allowed to become an end in itself, so it is worth indicating that a 'reasonable' level of body fat is positively necessary, especially when dealing with girls in the vulnerable teenage groups. 'Reasonable' here can be taken to be in the order of 18 per cent or more. In this author's experience, between 16 per cent and 18 per cent is the threshold body fat value below which many young women may well stop menstruating. This is not to suggest that the low body fat causes the periods to stop: indeed the amenorrhoea and the low fat level may share a common cause in the high level of training for elite competition performance.

It is known that amenorrhoea due to high levels of sporting activity may be associated with a degree of osteoporosis, or calcium loss from the bones, and this in turn may be linked with a higher risk of stress fractures. Thus one can make a good case for not allowing female teenagers, especially, to get too low in body fat or in body weight. A girl's training diary should keep a record of her periods, and if she has less than four periods in a year, medical advice should be sought. If it seems that a girl has sport-related amenorrhoea, it may be helpful to increase the daily calorie intake. The calcium intake is important, and this can be increased by taking a daily extra pint of low-fat milk, which contains about 600 mg of calcium, roughly half the day's requirement. The girl's doctor may suggest that she should take the contraceptive pill as a source of oestrogen, because a low oestrogen level can be the final link in the chain of causes of sporting amenorrhoea.

Their extra fat can be an advantage to girls. It gives them greater buoyancy and streamlining, so may well help them in swimming. Also it keeps them warmer under cold conditions, as in sea, lake and loch swimming, higher altitude and winter climbing, and sailing. On average, women are better sea and loch swimmers: for example, eight out of the ten fastest swims across the English Channel to date have been by women, and this is at least partly due to their better subcutaneous fat insulation. The fat increase at puberty is largely responsible for the changing shape of the female adolescent, a change which brings with it alterations to the centre of gravity both in the body and in individual limb segments. This may adversely influence some high-skill sports such as gymnastics, diving, trampolining, dance and ice-skating, all of which may have been taken up several years before puberty.

Many studies indicate the beneficial effects of exercise on blood fat levels in even relatively young children.[19, 20, 21] The high-density lipoproteins (HDL), which are considered beneficial, have been shown to be higher in children doing regular training.[19] It is also thought that the pattern for the development of atherosclerosis (furring up of the arteries) in adults may be laid down in the pre-pubescent years: the two factors thought to decrease the risk of coronary artery disease, a low blood level of triglycerides and high blood levels of high-density lipoproteins, were found to be correlated with participation in vigorous exercise in young children.[20] Blood lipid profiles were shown to benefit from regular exercise in a study which compared 12-year-old gymnasts, swimmers and unsporting girls, who were matched on the basis of sexual development. The gymnasts had the highest levels of the beneficial high-density lipoproteins, followed by the swimmers.[21]

This beneficial effect on blood fats is one of the most important reasons why children should be encouraged to develop early exercise habits which they can follow throughout life. While active sport and a balanced diet can control body fat levels to the accepted normal levels, parents should not be too insistent that their children, especially girls, be slim-looking.

Muscle strength

Strength is the ability of muscle to generate force. Force is proportional to the cross-sectional area of the muscle, and is modified and controlled by the nervous system (brain, spinal cord and associated motor nerves). Muscle exerts its force through tendons which anchor onto bones, which act as levers to magnify force or speed. As muscle becomes stronger, so do the tendons and the appropriate bones. Inadequate physical activity in children may hinder the normal development of the psychomotor and musculoskeletal system. A significant reduction of physical working capacity, including strength, may occur in hypo-active children upon reaching adulthood.[22] In other words, a child who does not take enough exercise risks being an under-strength adult.

For adults, at least part of their ability to become stronger involves the central nervous system's capacity to 'learn' to recruit a higher percentage of muscle fibres into relatively simultaneous contraction. Technically, this is the *neurogenic* aspect of strength gain. In children, this ability seems less pronounced. Their strength gains are related more to changes in the functioning of the muscle fibres themselves, technically called the *myogenic* component of strength. The two major aspects involved in children's strength gains are muscle protein synthesis and hypertrophy (enlargement).[14]

Strength is measured in the laboratory on specialized equipment which records the force developed in a whole range of movements and at different speeds. In the field, simple weightlifting tests may be used together with hand grip meters. An important attribute in sport is muscle power, which is a combination of the force and the speed with which the muscle may generate it. Sports coaches often talk of *strength-power* or *speed-power*, depending on which aspect is the more

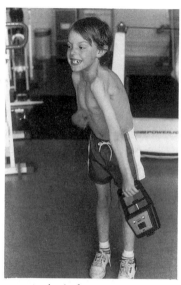

A grip dynamometer.

important for a given sport. For example, strength-power is important in the rugby scrum, and speed-power for throwing the javelin or for jumping. Putting the shot, on the other hand, is an example of a strength-power event for younger children (even though they use a lighter shot) which changes to a speed-power event for older competitors.

When children from 9 years old up to young adulthood were tested in the laboratory to measure the strength, contraction speed and fatigue in the lower leg calf muscles, soleus and gastrocnemius, it was found that contraction speed and fatigue resistance remained constant with increasing age, and did not differ according to the sex of the child. The strength remained the same in 9- to 11-year-old boys and girls, but after this phase, strength increased with age.

There is no doubt that strength increases naturally with growth, probably reaching a peak during the adolescent growth spurt in girls, and a year after the growth spurt in boys.[23] It has been suggested that suitable resistance training results in strength gains in girls throughout their phases of development, whether before puberty, at puberty or after it.[24] Similarly, boys too can improve their strength through training.[25, 26] There is some uncertainty as to whether strength trainability remains the same throughout the growth phases;[25]

whether pre-pubescents might have greater trainability in strength than older age groups;[24] or, on the contrary, whether older children have greater strength trainability than the pre-pubescents.[27] It has been questioned whether strength training in pre-adolescents is worthwhile, for example on the basis that three matched groups of 200 children aged 7 to 12, consisting of swimmers, tennis players or non-competitors, showed no differences in strength, except that the swimmers had better leg extension strength. However, none of the groups actually did any strength training, so the judgement was made on the basis of the presumed strength training contained in the actual sports.[28]

Boys tend to have fairly large increases in strength after puberty, when the anabolic effect of their testicular hormones triggers hypertrophy in the muscle mass, which is already increasing through normal growth. Girls do not have such a marked increase following puberty, although they do produce some anabolic androgens from their adrenal glands, and some of their ovarian hormone has an anabolic effect. Girls tend to have a more gradual rise in strength from a younger age than boys, and in part this may be due to their muscle being more sensitive to the effects of growth hormone, which is present throughout childhood. Indeed, this has led to claims that girls are more responsive to strength training before puberty than are boys.

When discussing strength training for children, it is important to appreciate that there is a big difference between weight training and the sport of weightlifting. In weightlifting, the aim is to achieve a maximal lift, the greatest possible weight one can move in a given pattern, usually once only at a time. In weight training for general conditioning, a lighter load is moved several times, usually at least ten up to approximately twenty times: this is called submaximal resistance training, and the weight is never too heavy to lift correctly over the chosen number of repetitions. The American Academy of Pediatrics has issued a strong caution about the potential dangers of weightlifting for children,[29] and it has been said that weightlifting for the growing child 'should be considered damaging, unless proven otherwise'.[30] It is therefore disappointing that weightlifters and powerlifters can compete from very young ages.

While weight training with light loading may be beneficial for the young sports player, and may be necessary for remedial exercises following injury, any kind of heavy resistance training should be avoided until full bone growth has been achieved. It is known that children are capable of learning sports skills from the age of 6, but it is thought that they do not appreciate or understand the value of systematic, planned training programmes until 11 or 12 at the earliest; therefore 13 to 14 could be considered the youngest age group suitable for concentrated programmes.[31] Even then, heavy squats, extensor thrusts against resistance and plyometric jumping, if overdone, may produce a high incidence of damage, including bone injuries. The precocious elite child competitor in particular sports, such as gymnastics, swimming and tennis may have a considerable appetite for strength training: such training should be carefully monitored in terms of quantity and quality, and should be very modestly progressive. In particular, the coach should be very alert to the child's indication of any pain, especially persistent or crescendo pain, associated with strength training.

Muscle endurance (anaerobic fitness)

The ability to perform repeated muscle movements, as in rowing, canoeing or running upstairs, may be referred to as *local muscle endurance*. Such endurance often has a high anaerobic energy component. Muscle has two main sources of energy, an *aerobic* supply which needs oxygen, and an *anaerobic* supply (meaning literally 'without air'), which is brought in for major efforts whose energy demands exceed the aerobic supply. Anaerobic energy is derived directly and solely from glucose or glycogen (the form in which glucose is stored) in muscle cells. Anaerobic work occurs in two ways: either as short continuous activity such as 400-metre running, or longer intermittent work as in canoeing or rowing. *Anaerobic power* is the rate at which the work is done without oxygen. *Anaerobic capacity* is a person's total capability for a single sustained bout of anaerobic work, whether it is a longer intermittent series, as in rowing, or a shorter continuous effort, as in sprinting. The by-product of anaerobic work is lactic acid, which leads to rising fatigue and muscle pain. The *anaerobic threshold* is the level of exercise at which lactic acid begins to accumulate in the blood. Younger children have a significantly lower ability to work anaerobically compared to adolescents, who themselves are inferior in this respect to adults.

Tests used to assess *anaerobic power* and the *local muscle endurance* of children include the very useful Wingate Anaerobic Test, devised by Oded Bar-Or. The child works a cycle ergometer using legs or arms as hard as possible for thirty seconds against a work load which is calculated as a proportion of the child's body weight. This test can be used for children as young as 5.[32] Usually the test is computerized to record the speed of the flywheel and the load, and to calculate the peak level of anaerobic power produced, together with the rate of fatigue. Anaerobic capacity is probably best estimated by a post-exercise oxygen consumption test (i.e. oxygen debt): for instance, the subject may exercise at maximum effort in the laboratory for two or three minutes, and the 'extra' oxygen used, above the amount needed to sustain the resting metabolism, is measured over the subsequent ten minutes. The bigger the oxygen 'debt', the better the anaerobic capacity. A simple field test for small children consists of asking them to perform half squat (knee bend) movements, which are counted over a given time to test the quadriceps muscles on the front of the thigh; the calf muscles can be tested similarly by asking the child to go up and down on his or her toes as many times as possible in the given time.[33]

Even when allowances are made for differences in bodyweight, the anaerobic energy produced by an 8-year-old is only 70 per cent of that of an 11-year-old, which in turn is less than that of a 14-year-old.[34] I would deny that these differences are simply due to the younger children having poorer motivation when under test, as has been suggested. The younger child's muscle has less glycogen, and a much lower rate of utilization of glycogen, and it has less creatine-phosphate, the immediate anaerobic energy store.[35a] It has also been shown that children have lower maximal concentrations of lactic acid in blood and muscle at various high percentages of maximum effort, compared to adults undergoing similar levels of exercise stress.[36, 37, 38] Young children have a distinctly lower mechanical power output than adolescents and young adults, both absolutely and relatively, when assessed by the Margaria step-running test.[36] On the Wingate test, leg power in children has been shown to increase with age and to go on increasing until the end of the third decade, whereas arm power, similarly measured, reaches its highest value at the end of the second decade.

At the beginning of exercise, energy is derived anaerobically for about the first half-minute, and this deficit has to be repaid more or less immediately by energy from aerobic sources. Exercise always feels particularly hard just before this deficit is paid, but immediately

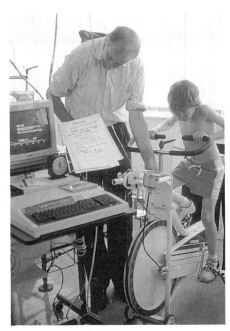

The Wingate test.

afterwards one works more easily: this is called getting a *second wind*. At the end of a period of strenuous exercise one goes on breathing very heavily for some minutes. This may be referred to as repaying the *oxygen debt*. The oxygen debt is due mainly to the need to replenish depleted energy stores. Children incur less of an oxygen deficit at the beginning of exercise,[39] which implies that they gain their 'second wind' earlier than adults. Also, their capacity to incur an 'oxygen debt' is less than that of adults, and their 'anaerobic threshold' is much higher. This is a major reason why many children seem able to be constantly active in situations where adults would suffer fatigue which would force them to ease off their activity level periodically.

It has been well documented that in children from 10 to 15 years, all their anaerobic parameters may be increased with training.[36, 38, 40] Anaerobic function may be investigated by doing appropriate laboratory tests before and after periods of training. Such tests may be measures of lactic acid in blood, or estimations of anaerobic power by the Wingate test, or levels of anaerobic capacity by oxygen debt assessment. One study evaluated the effect of a nine-week interval training programme on anaerobic parameters and the anaerobic threshold in 10- to 11-year-old boys.[41] The training increased the children's peak power output by 14 per cent, and the average power sustained over thirty seconds by 10 per cent. There was also a significant increase in running speed at the anaerobic threshold, although in relative terms (i.e., as a percentage of the maximum oxygen intake), the threshold declined by 4 per cent. The maximum oxygen intake increased by 8 per cent, taking bodyweight into account. Conclusions drawn from this study were that anaerobic threshold measures are less sensitive indicators of fitness levels than maximum oxygen intake in pre-adolescent boys, and that appropriate training may improve both maximum aerobic power and anaerobic capacity in this age group.

The great majority of the work on anaerobic aspects of children shows that they are much less anaerobic, and consequently more aerobic, than their older counterparts, and even more so than the fully adult. This would seem to suggest that their ideal activities should be modestly long as well as short. For instance, running middle distance events such as the 800 and 1500 metres may be just as suitable for children as sprints between 50 and 200 metres. For very young children, however, one has to remember that distances which appear short to adults seem a very long way, so that a 50-metre run may be an aerobic distance for a 5-year-old. Children are well adapted to relatively long periods of moderate physical activity, but they need appropriately frequent short rest periods, because they have fewer natural metabolic boundaries (such as high lactic acid levels), and can therefore over-heat and dehydrate. While young children are likely to be relatively more successful in longer distance exercise, in terms of running times, it is also advisable to include exercise involving faster, shorter bursts of activity for them, as their anaerobic parameters can be improved through training. This is especially relevant for the child whose main interest is in sports involving sharp bursts of activity, such as football, hockey or squash.

Aerobic fitness

The normal source of energy for moderate daily activity is supplied aerobically as muscle uses oxygen to release its fuel energy. The oxygen is absorbed from the air in the lungs. The air itself is drawn down the ever-smaller tubes (*bronchi*) of the bronchial tree, leading through the smallest bronchioles into the air sacs (*alveoli*) where the oxygen is taken up and carbon dioxide given off. The bronchi have muscular walls and are capable of active constriction and passive dilation. On diffusing through the alveolar walls, the oxygen is taken into the alveolar capillaries and carried by the chemical *haemoglobin* in the red cells of the blood down ever-smaller arteries, until it reaches the capillaries. The capillaries are the finest twigs of the vascular tree, and they lie in direct contact with all cells, including muscle cells. In the muscle cells, another similar chemical, *myoglobin*, is responsible for transporting the oxygen deep into the cell to the thousands of tiny *mitochondria*, which are the sites where the oxygen is used to release energy from fat or glucose, the cell's aerobic fuels.

During exercise, the volume of air ventilated by the lungs may increase by ten- to twenty-fold, while there may be a five-fold increase in the output of blood from the heart. The heart may increase its rate of beating (the *pulse rate*) by two or three times, and it may nearly double the amount of blood pumped at each beat (the *stroke volume*). The pumping causes the blood to be under pressure in the blood vessels. This pressure is higher just as the heart beats (the *systolic pressure*), and lower in between beats (the *diastolic pressure*). This is why blood pressure readings are usually given as two figures, such as 120/80, which refer to the systolic and diastolic pressures respectively, and are usually measured in millimetres of mercury (mmHg) using a sphygmomanometer.

Sudden death. Heart-associated deaths during activity, exercise or sport usually involve *sudden death*, and can happen without any obvious warning signs. The causes of such sudden death fall mainly into three categories: congenital, where the heart is malformed (various types of malformation are possible, some of which are compatible with strenuous exercise, up to a point); infectious, in which some viruses and the toxins from some bacteria may damage the heart, during or just after the illness; and pathological, where a condition such as atherosclerosis (chronic inflammation of arteries, including the coronary arteries in the heart) may lead to deposition of fatty material inside the arteries, causing a great reduction in blood flow and a potential for blockage. Children may suffer from congenital or infectious categories. The former should be diagnosed early in life, but in some cases heart malformation is hard to detect, especially if there is no particular reason for suspecting it. Regarding the second, children (and adults) should simply not undertake very strenuous activity until some days after any illness which has involved a fever (i.e., a raised temperature and pulse rate), particularly if it has been bad enough to need bed-rest for a day or more. Specific conditions, such as rheumatic and glandular fever, are well known to cause possible damage to the heart, sometimes requiring months or, in the case of rheumatic fever, even years of lay-off from strenuous activity.

Children's breathing. The capillaries, myoglobin and the mitochondria may all be increased by appropriate training, in all age groups. Increases in a child's lung volume, however, are entirely due to the growth in body dimensions: they are not dependent on increases in physical performance capacity.[42] Children breathe much faster than adults during exercise, taking shorter and shallower breaths. Where an adult, for example, may have a respiratory rate of forty breaths per minute during exercise, a child's rate may be sixty. Technically, the amount of air needed to give one litre of oxygen is called the *ventilatory equivalent*. The younger the child, the more litres of air have to be breathed in to obtain one litre of oxygen. The 6-year-old child may need to breathe in thirty-eight litres of air to

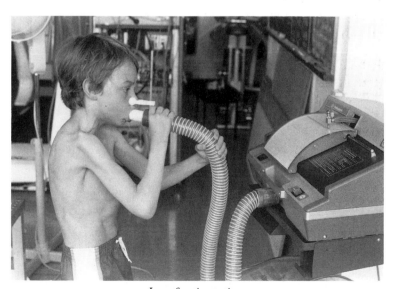

Lung function testing.

gain one litre of oxygen, whereas the ventilatory equivalent for an 18-year-old in similar conditions may be only twenty-eight litres.[35b]

It is not harmful that the child has to breathe in more air to gain necessary oxygen, but it is wasteful of energy in terms of the extra muscular work required for the breathing, and it is also wasteful of body water. It *may* also be one cause of 'contagious hysteria', when groups of children panic as a response to the feelings of dizziness and lightheadedness caused when they blow off too much carbon dioxide, for instance after a prolonged singing session. Breathing out too much carbon dioxide is technically called *hyperventilation hypocapnia*, and it can also lead to cramp-like contractions of the hands and feet, together with numbness around the mouth. One cure for it is to breathe in and out of a medium-sized paper bag for periods of about ten seconds at a time, thus re-breathing expired carbon dioxide to redress the balance of gases in the respiratory system.

Very cold or dry air also causes constriction of the lung airways in everyone who exercises strenuously in cold winter weather, for instance outside on a cold pitch or field, or inside in an unheated squash court or gymnasium. At worst, the cold air may provoke an asthmatic attack in a child who has the condition, or it may induce or worsen exercise-induced asthma. Therefore, you should take special care of children exercising in the cold, particularly if they are known to have asthma. The child with exercise-induced asthma may need to use an inhaler before sport on cold days, and may need reminding of this. Provided the condition is well controlled, there is no reason for an asthmatic child not to do sport, even in cold weather. If a child has a sudden asthmatic attack, he or she should be taken to the doctor as quickly as possible. While transport is being organized, or during the journey, the child should be encouraged to sit comfortably, resting elbows on knees, and to do controlled breathing exercises, particularly concentrating on breathing out, in order to take better breaths in.

Smoking. As might be expected, little work has been done on the effect of cigarette smoking on children's fitness. However, many young people do smoke, so you should be aware of the possible consequences. Tobacco smoking has both short-term (acute) and long-term (chronic) effects which are potentially harmful. The possible long-term effects include bronchial cancer, chronic bronchitis and an increased risk of heart attack, among other serious conditions. The many short-term effects have an adverse influence on aerobic performance.

There are two main acute effects of smoking, one caused by the carbon or soot particles, and the other by the carbon monoxide in the smoke. Simply, the smoke particles irritate the epithelial lining of the bronchi in the lung. The bronchi respond partly by constricting, thus narrowing the airways, and partly by producing more mucus to assist in the removal of the soot particles. However, the extra mucus also contributes to the airway narrowing, and the net result is to cut down the flow of air into and out of the lung by around 10–15 per cent. The second acute effect of smoking is for the carbon monoxide gas present in tobacco smoke selectively to block oxygen from being carried by the haemoglobin of the red blood cells. Two cigarettes in an hour will effectively inactivate about 8 per cent of the oxygen-carrying capacity of the blood. This is a severe handicap in strenuous aerobic sports such as running, swimming, squash, hockey, shinty, lacrosse, soccer or rugby.

Passive smoking has similar, though lesser effects. Young children are at particular risk from passive smoking for two reasons. First, they are especially vulnerable to air pollutants because of the relatively greater amount of air (by up to 25 per cent) they have to inspire per unit of bodyweight. Second, infants and toddlers are captive audiences of smoking parents, especially their mothers. Five-year-old children of mothers who smoke have lungs which may be only 90 per cent of their expected volume. If children of smoking parents smoke themselves, even very moderately, their lung development may decrease further. If you are an adult smoker, you should be aware of the harmful effect of your habit on young sports players. If you are driving children to a competition or practice facility, for instance, you should try to avoid smoking in the car. You should also try to keep children away from smoky atmospheres, for instance in a club house or refreshment area. Even outdoors, you should avoid smoking near children, as the smoke may not be dissipated quickly and they can still inhale it.

The limiting effects of smoking on exercise capacity may not be noticed during ordinary everyday activities. The effects may not reduce performance in sports involving short impulses or bursts of intense exercise, such as jumping, throwing or sprinting. However, smoking has a marked and noticeable effect on performance in any form of continuous strenuous exercise or sport which lasts longer than two or three minutes. If children or teenagers have already developed a smoking habit, despite participating in sports, the very *least* you can give by way of advice is to ask them not to smoke for a minimum of four hours before doing any sport, whether recreational or competitive. This gives time for the lung airways and the blood to restore themselves to a reasonable level of normality. Children should always be discouraged from smoking, and encouraged to give up if they do become addicted.

Heart rates. Maximal heart rates for both sexes are about 200 per minute at the age of 20, roughly following the formula that the age-related maximum heart rate is equal to 220 minus the age in years. Children's maximum heart rates may well reach 215 or more, but they are unlikely to reach such high levels once maturity has been reached. These higher rates may compensate for the relatively small heart size in children. At proportionately equal exercise loads, a child's heart may well beat at twenty per minute more than an adult's, and at lower blood pressure.

When blood pressure (p. 48) measurements were made in 500 healthy 9- to 18-year-olds during dynamic exercise, it was found that systolic blood pressure increased more in the post-pubertal groups than in those who had not yet reached puberty. Twenty-two children reached a systolic pressure of 200 mmHg, with three post-pubertal boys reaching 240 mmHg at heart rates of 170, blood pressure levels which the researcher considered inadvisable.[43] In this author's laboratory, systolic pressures of over 400 mmHg have been recorded in adult wrestlers. A separate study of ice-skaters between 9 and 14 years of age showed that their diastolic pressure decreased significantly at maximal exercise, as compared to a separate control group of children.[44] This was interpreted as indicating that the skaters, who all trained for at least fifteen hours per week, had better adaptation of their peripheral blood vessel system to the demands of exercise. In adults, of course, appropriate aerobic exercise has been shown to be associated with a general lowering of the blood pressure, so it may be beneficial to initiate this process early in life.

It has been suggested that different forms of enlargement of the heart (cardiac hypertrophy) follow from different modes of training.[45, 46] For example, isotonic or dynamic exercise, such as running, swimming, cycling, football, hockey, lacrosse or squash, could be associated with large hearts with relatively unthickened walls, if performed at high levels during childhood. On the other hand, 'strength' sports, or those linked with more static forms of training, such as weightlifting, weight training, gymnastics, rowing or canoeing, might produce smaller hearts with relatively thicker walls. Speculation has centred on whether such thicker-walled hearts might not be associated with higher blood pressure in later life. However, considerable doubt exists as to whether the heart really responds so differently to training.[47, 48] No evidence has been found that child competitors eventually develop larger hearts in later life than other athletes who did not begin competitive sport in early childhood.[48] It has been suggested that intensive dynamic training promotes a real increase in left ventricular mass, together with an absolute increase in heart volume.[48]

Static or isometric muscle work is associated with greater rises in blood pressure than muscle work of lower intensity but in which there is frequent movement, such as running, swimming and skipping. This is why heavy lifting, digging, snow-shovelling or push-starting cars are inadvisable activities for adults whose blood pressure is known to be already high. A rapid progress in cardiac dilatation and hypertrophy may occur in response to only a few months of intensive dynamic training, with a corresponding regression once the training has stopped, not only in adults, but also in children before the age of puberty.[48]

A study which investigated the electrocardiograph changes in fifty 10- to 11-year-old boys of varying fitness levels, after both endurance and short anaerobic modes of exercise, showed no changes which could be related to growth or fitness status.[49] There have been few studies of the relationship between stroke volume (p. 48) and heart rate in children, but one showed that the stroke volume in a group of 11-year-olds was greatest at heart rates of between 100 and 120 beats per minute.[50] Because of this, it has been suggested that moderate continuous exercise at these heart rates might be the optimal form of training for the heart in younger children. This is contrary to the current thinking on adult aerobic training, where the consensus seems to be moving towards performing higher intensity work to initiate a training effect on the heart (but lower, longer work to effect aerobic changes in muscle).

The question of what effect the early training influence in childhood has on ultimate cardiac development in much later life is a very important one, and needs much more in the way of long-term studies. However, as it is known that aerobic exercise can improve capillary and muscle function and can help prevent the atherosclerosis which can begin even in pre-pubescent years, there can be little doubt that appropriate early exercise or activity habits are very important for the young child.

Aerobic fitness tests. The quantity of oxygen used in a given time is termed *aerobic power*. Aerobic power depends on the ability of the lungs to take in the air; on the blood to absorb the oxygen from the lungs; on the heart to deliver adequate quantities of blood to the muscles; and finally on the muscles' ability to utilize the oxygen to release the food energy. The more it uses oxygen, the more a muscle generates energy. For each litre of oxygen used by a muscle, approximately five kilocalories (22.5 kJ) of energy are released. For a given volume of oxygen utilized, more energy is released from glycogen and glucose than fat (as free fatty acids) in muscle. When aerobic fitness is measured, bodyweight is taken into account and the oxygen uptake ($\dot{V}O_2$ max) results are *normalized*, that is expressed per kilogram of bodyweight: otherwise heavier children would always tend to have the highest values. (Nevertheless, such normalized values may themselves give misleading results due to the spurious nature of some biological ratio standards especially regarding the correlation of indices.)[51, 52] Oxygen uptake values are expressed as millilitres (ml) of oxygen (O_2) per kilogram of bodyweight (kg) per minute (min), technically abbreviated to $ml.O_2kg^{-1}.min^{-1}$. Between the ages of 5 and 10 years, aerobic power is similar in both sexes. Due to their earlier growth spurts, girls may then go ahead, but from about 14 onwards their aerobic power tends not to improve relatively, mainly because of their increase in body fat percentage at this stage of development. Boys, on the other hand, continue to improve their aerobic power until the age of 18.

There are many different methods of testing children for aerobic power. Some tests use sophisticated modern equipment in a laboratory, whereas simpler tests can be done in the field. The important aspect of all testing, but particularly 'field' testing, is that the subject should be compared to his or her previous results, rather than being compared with the standard of other members of the group.[53] It should be said that children's tests show great variance in their results, and a large part of the differences can be accounted for by differences in age, stage of maturation, height, weight, sex, somatotype (body structure), level of training, and especially by motivation.[54] Therefore valid comparisons between children in a group are difficult to make.

A typical maximum oxygen uptake ($\dot{V}O_2$ max) for 12.8-year-olds would be 47.8 ml.kg^{-1}.min^{-1} for boys, and 39.5 for girls.[55] For 16- to 19-year-olds, a study on 270 adolescents revealed aerobic power values of 51.7 ml.kg^{-1}.min^{-1} for the boys, and 40.0 for the girls.[56] These results were all obtained on the treadmill, which tends to produce values around 5 per cent higher than cycle tests. Some workers have measured children from the age of 4 upwards, and have noted that different treadmill protocols produce much the same maximum oxygen uptake values.[57, 58, 59] On the more elite side of performance, a study on club and County standard runners specializing in 800 metres up to 3000 metres showed that the boys recorded mean $\dot{V}O_2$ max values of 70.0 ml.kg^{-1}.min^{-1}, while the girls recorded 64.0 ml.kg^{-1}.min^{-1}.[60]

The multistage 20-metre shuttle run test (20-MST) is a simpler test of aerobic fitness than treadmill testing, but it is still effective. In

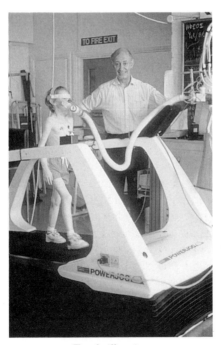

Treadmill testing.

the 20-MST, subjects run back and forth at increasing speeds, starting from 8.5 km.hr^{-1}, and changing speed according to a sound signal. When the subject can no longer follow the pace, the final speed reached is used to predict maximum oxygen uptake. The 20-MST is a reasonably accurate test of maximal aerobic power.[61, 62] A modified version has been developed in the author's laboratory for use on the squash court.[63]

A less effective test is the six-minute endurance run. A study comparing this test with the treadmill found that the results failed to correlate accurately.[62] For physical education classes, it has been suggested that children can be roughly classified into endurance categories on the basis of testing them with a 600-metre run for those aged 9 or less, a 1500-metre or nine-minute run for children aged 10 to 13, and a 2500-metre or twelve-minute run for older adolescents.[64]

This author has found a version of the Step-Test to be a useful field measure in confined situations. I used it, for instance, for the England boys' squash squads, whose age-groups ranged from

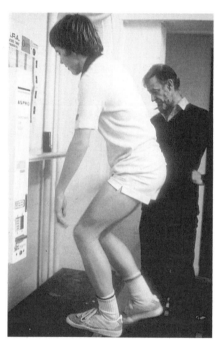

'Field testing': the Step-Test.

under-10 to under-19, and whose physiological tests were mainly done in corridors or other spaces around the squash courts. Step heights of 14 to 18 inches (36 to 46 cm) and cadences of twenty to thirty steps per minute were used according to the age, size and height of the boys.

The *anaerobic threshold* is a term much used in the exercise testing of adults because it can be a very useful measure, oddly enough, of the level of *aerobic* exercise which can be maintained for a reasonable length of time. When you do graded exercise, there is a point at which the exercise becomes so hard that there is a disproportionate rise in your pulmonary ventilation, heart rate, or blood lactic acid, in relation to the increase in oxygen uptake. The anaerobic threshold can be defined as the oxygen uptake which occurs immediately below this level. The three important parameters have technical terms relating to this level of exercise: the pulmonary ventilation rise can be termed the *ventilation threshold*, the heart rate level is called the *cardiac threshold*, and the lactic acid increase is the *lactate threshold* or *onset of blood lactate accumulation* (OBLA). It is currently assumed that training at immediately sub-anaerobic threshold levels is the most efficient way of improving aerobic fitness. When the anaerobic threshold is measured, the physiologist can advise the athlete exactly what type and intensity of exercise to do in order to gain maximum aerobic training benefit. However, relatively little work has been done on children in this respect.

The anaerobic threshold can be determined by blood lactic acid or blood gas analyses during aerobic testing.[65, 66] A much simpler but less effective method is to use heart rate or breathing measures. One study showed that the ventilation threshold of 11-year-old boys tested on a cycle ergometer occurred at 58 per cent of their maximal oxygen uptake.[67] Another study of 257 boys and girls aged 5.7 to 15.5 years showed that the ventilation threshold decreased with age, and that there were only low correlations between the threshold and maximum oxygen uptake, in contrast to the results of studies on adults.[68] Metabolic systems in sporting children have to respond to two dynamic processes relating to growth *and* training respectively. It has been noted that children have a disproportionate growth of their cardiorespiratory system, compared to their metabolic function.[69]

Trainability. One often hears reference to increasing a child's or young person's 'stamina'. Stamina, endurance, or 'staying power' is the capacity for sustained aerobic exercise using a high proportion of the maximum oxygen uptake ($\dot{V}O_2$ max), whatever its level.[70] However, the child's level of stamina only partly involves aerobic fitness as defined, for it also depends in part on the child's degree of motivation. The levels of fitness and motivation are both very important in all forms of prolonged endurance exercise for children. In general, the younger the child, the more important is motivation as a component of 'stamina', not least when one is conducting fitness tests. Children involved in competitive sport tend, almost by definition, to be more highly motivated in endurance situations, whether in training, competition, or in field or laboratory tests.

There is currently much debate on the trainability of various parameters of children's fitness. It has been shown that specific endurance training can improve the $\dot{V}O_2$ max as well as the aerobic threshold in boys aged between 9 and 11.[71] Physical activity at moderate to high intensity in pre-pubescent children seems to increase $\dot{V}O_2$ max, rather than the lactate threshold.[72] This is indeed what one might expect, given the lower propensity to lactate production of children in this age group. A 'law of quantity' has been formulated: the higher the ability level, the more one has to practise.[73] This indicates that from puberty onwards, the trainer or physical educator has to differentiate stress loads, particularly with respect to ability level.

Data on maximal aerobic power in normal children, trained and untrained, from 4 to 16 years have been reviewed.[74] Training programmes certainly increase both relative and absolute $\dot{V}O_2$ max in both sexes, although no specific year can be pinpointed as the one in which training will show the greatest benefit. In a study on elite competitors aged 15 to 20, it was shown that the heart adapted functionally up to 15 to 17 years, but thereafter the increase in the amount and intensity of training significantly accelerated the growth of the heart.[75] Interestingly, from changes in oxidative enzymes, it was suggested that muscle in the 15 to 17 age group may respond better to training than muscle in older age groups. It is already thought that adults may need relatively higher intensity training to affect the cardiorespiratory–haemic axis, but relatively lower intensity and longer training to affect the oxygen distribution and utilization systems within the muscles. From the research just quoted, it is possible that mid- to late-teenagers may respond similarly.

A high intensity exercise programme, when the heart rate was raised to a mean level of 177 beats per minute, was found to result in significant improvements in the aerobic power of a group of 9-year-olds.[76] Some training programmes produce little or no improvement in children's $\dot{V}O_2$ max, but it is probable that these programmes are simply not hard enough. Even in pre-pubescent children, it has been found that high intensity training sessions, reaching heart rates of 60 per cent to 90 per cent of the maximum, have to be done for at least fifteen minutes, three to five times per week, in order to improve $\dot{V}O_2$ max beyond the normal rate of improvement with age.[77] The current author, like other researchers,[78] believes that adult training regimes are not appropriate until the end of the adolescent growth spurt.

Altitude training is used by many competitors, especially in the longer aerobic events, although there is still much controversy over whether it can provide an increase in top-class sea-level performance. I believe that altitude training can give the elite competitor a small but important boost. There is much less doubt that altitude training may benefit appropriate competitors of club level ability. I know of no comparable work which has been done on children and altitude training. Like adults, children acclimatize to altitude, so presumably they might benefit from appropriate altitude training. One should remember that the human foetus is effectively living at high altitude while in the uterus: its oxygen supply is equivalent to that at 23,000 feet (7,000 metres), and it has a special form of haemoglobin to cope with this, which is gradually replaced some months later, after birth.

One factor worth noting is that deficiencies in vitamin C, riboflavin (vitamin B_2) and pyridoxin (B_6) in a group of 12- to 15-year-olds correlated with decreased working capacity. Once the deficiencies were corrected, $\dot{V}O_2$ max levels rose correspondingly.[79] This emphasizes the importance of a properly balanced diet for physical fitness.

In summary:
- Older children are higher in absolute levels of aerobic power than younger children, progressively so with age. However, when adjustments are made to allow for the differences in bodyweight between the younger and older children, the $\dot{V}O_2$ max results show much less difference between the age groups.
- After puberty the relative and absolute $\dot{V}O_2$ max levels increase in

boys, whereas they decline in girls, or at least show lower levels of increase.

- All children gain a higher proportion of their energy from aerobic than anaerobic sources, compared to adults.
- Anaerobic thresholds and $\dot{V}O_2$ max levels may be increased with training at all ages, although more effectively at the end of the growth spurt.
- Atherosclerotic disease in the blood vessels may start in pre-teenage children; thus it is particularly important to begin good dietary and exercise habits as early as possible.
- Children should, of course, be very strongly discouraged from smoking.
- Strenuous exercise in cold winter conditions may induce or worsen asthma in vulnerable children.
- Motivation is a particularly important component of fitness testing.
- It is essential for children (like adults) not to exercise when ill, or suffering from any kind of infection, or too soon after any illness requiring bed-rest.

Movement economy. The amount of oxygen needed for a particular activity or set of movements, termed the *oxygen cost*, is part of what is known as *movement economy*. This is increasingly being perceived as an important factor in fatigue, especially in association with running. There is significant variation in running economy, or the oxygen cost of running at a given speed, between children and adults, and important differences may be found even within a group of elite distance runners.[80] Children are 'wasteful' of energy in running, not only through their biomechanics but also for biochemical reasons: they have lower stores of muscle glycogen and lower concentrations of appropriate muscle enzymes. The oxygen costs of walking and running are higher in children than in adults.[81] Young children use more oxygen than older age groups.[82] Children with more efficient movement economy have better stamina, and can keep running at the same pace for longer than those with a high oxygen cost.[83] It has also been noted that running economy in teenage girls improves not only with age, but also with training.[84]

Possible causes of the lower degree of running economy in children are complex. It seems likely that it is the biomechanical aspects of running which create the great differences between the age-groups. In cycling, on the other hand, the energy costs for younger and older children, and for adults, are much closer for a given workload, suggesting that the intrinsic aerobic metabolic efficiency of muscle at the various ages is similar. In children there may be a marked improvement in distance running during periods when the $\dot{V}O_2$ max remains the same.[60] One possible explanation might be that children are not kinetically balanced, and economy of effort is sacrificed for speed.

A further cause of children's lower running economy may lie in their energy storage capacity in terms of elastic strain energy in the leg tendons, especially the Achilles tendon, and in the ligaments of the arches of the foot. The recovery and re-utilization of elastic strain energy has a very marked effect on the economy of rebound movement[85] and of running.[80, 86] Again, it may be the case that lighter children are not kinetically balanced in terms of optimal weight loading of the visco-elastic structures of their limbs during striding. It remains true that young children are capable of impressive achievements in distance running, like the 7-year-old boy who completed the full-distance marathon race in just over three and a half hours:[3] the current author believes the boy should not have been encouraged to do the marathon, but the feat is undoubtedly very great.

Practical applications arising from these considerations of children's running economy include:

1. The importance of attending to running style in younger athletes.
2. The importance of not using adult fitness equations for children: for instance, the Cooper twelve-minute-run test equation can be replaced by the age-specific MacDougal equation.[87]
3. The need to realize that young children may be working much harder than they appear to be during a wide variety of activities, from squash to hill walking, and that family cycling would be easier on children than strenuous long walks.

Flexibility and mobility

Very few good data are available on the development of flexibility and mobility during childhood. The child's ability to move his or her joints through degrees of movement depends partly on genetic factors, and partly on the amount of movement the joints are put through on a regular basis. A joint's range of motion is limited by the joint structure itself: that is the way the bone ends meet, the shape of the bones, the tightness of the binding capsule, and the strength of the retaining ligaments. It is also limited by the length of the muscles which surround and control it. To distinguish between these two components in movement range, it is usual to refer to *mobility* in relation to joint movement, and *flexibility* in relation to muscle elasticity, although there have been other suggestions for describing joint motion.[88]

The body's joints are designed with different ranges and directions of movement, according to their function. The shoulder joint, for instance, is a ball-and-socket joint loosely bound within its capsule to allow maximum freedom of movement between the bones. This allows us to reach up above our head, or round behind our back. The hip joint, by contrast, although also a ball-and-socket joint, is firmly held by a relative negative pressure inside its capsule. The bones are held in close congruity by an extremely strong central ligament, and the joint is surrounded by tough ligaments, tendons and muscles. Although the hip's movements are similar to the shoulder's, the amount of range is relatively limited, to give the joint maximum stability. The elbow joint is a pure hinge, capable of bending and straightening, whereas the knee is a more complex condylar joint, able not only to bend and straighten, but also to twist inwards and outwards to a certain degree.

The amount of movement that can be produced voluntarily in any given joint is called the *active range* of movement. Apart from the joint's natural limitations, its active movement may be limited by muscle weakness, muscle tightness or joint stiffness perhaps caused by injury, lack of use or fatigue. Sitting still for long periods, for example, causes joint stiffness partly because the joints' synovial fluid lubricates them less effectively, and partly because of muscle shortening. The *passive range* of movement is the degree of motion obtained through external pressure, for instance if the physiologist moves the joint through its full range and presses it into the stretched position. All the bones in moving joints can also be moved in directions which cannot be achieved actively, but only by passive manipulation. There are called *accessory movements*, and automatically form part of a joint's normal movements. The head of the humerus can be glided backwards and forwards within the shoulder joint capsule, for instance. If the accessory movements are impaired for any reason, they limit a joint's overall mobility.

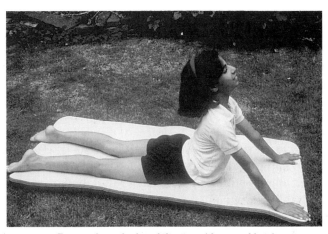

Extreme lower back mobility in a 10-year-old girl.

A child may have very loose, mobile joints. This is technically called *hypermobility*. The elbows and knees might curve backwards when the joints are straightened. The child may be able to touch the thumb to the forearm on the same side, or bend the trunk backwards to place the head between the knees. It is unusual for all the joints to be hypermobile in all directions: more commonly certain joints are relatively stiff. For instance a child with a hypermobile lumbar spine and an exaggerated lordosis may not be able to stretch the arms upwards fully. Hypermobility is more common in girls than in boys. It can be an advantage in sports like gymnastics which require a high degree of flexibility. Young gymnasts and dancers often create hypermobility in joints, especially in the ankles and feet, through their training. However, hypermobility can contribute to injuries, especially in the teenage years and later, if the child does not gain sufficient strength in the lax muscles to stabilize and protect the joints.

It is well known that flexibility in general decreases with growth. This is most marked during growth spurts, when the increased length of the bones stretches the attached muscles over the bones: for a period, the muscles appear comparatively thin, until they gain strength and bulk.[89] If the child is involved in a sport which tends to shorten certain muscles, they tighten, altering joint range of movement. Many young elite squash players, for instance, gradually lose the ability to straighten their knees fully, due to the crouching stance of the game. Poor flexibility is, in itself, thought to be an important cause of overuse injuries.[90, 91] An imbalance between muscle strength and flexibility after a growth spurt, caused by failure to do flexibility training, or through doing sports which create muscle strength and tightness, is an important potential cause of muscle injury[92, 93, 94] and, directly or indirectly, of joint injury.[95]

Joint range can be measured in certain cases with a goniometer, an instrument which calculates the degree of flexion (bend) or extension the joint can achieve. The sit-and-reach test measures hamstring flexibility, and can include the lower and middle back. Monitoring children's flexibility can be done in many different ways, so the physiologist, coach or physiotherapist doing the measuring should always record how the child has been positioned, and how the measurements have been taken. If possible, the same person should perform the measurements each time the child is monitored.

There are also various methods of improving mobility and flexibility.[96] Mobilizing exercises (often called *ballistic exercises*) involve rapid repetitive movements which gradually increase joint movement range. Repetitive toe-touching or trunk side-bending movements are examples of these. This type of exercise is most suitable for very young (pre-teen) children. It is effective in loosening the joint structures and improving joint fluid lubrication. However, it carries a strong risk of over-stretching the muscles in older children, because the elastic limit of the moving muscles can easily be exceeded.[97] Static or passive stretching is generally considered to be the safest and most suitable form of flexibility training for all age groups. The child stands, sits or lies so that the relevant muscles are placed in their longest comfortable position, and held still for a count of six to ten. The stretch is then released, and repeated, perhaps three to five times: there is usually a slight increase in flexibility each time.

There is some controversy about the correct way to do passive, Yoga-style stretching. Stretching wrongly, or over-stretching, can cause injuries.[98] It is vital for the child to learn to feel the limit of the stretch for each muscle group. The child should never hold the stretch for a long period, and then try to stretch further without relaxing first. Passive stretching exercises apply mainly to the arms and legs: for teenagers as for adults back problems can be caused by trying to stretch the spine. Equally, the child should not see stretching exercises as a challenge: children should not compete to

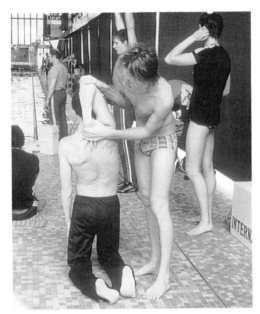

Advanced stretching techniques for elite swimmers.

stretch further than each other, nor should they be thinking about how far then can go. The very flexible child may do assisted passive stretching, with another person holding the arm or leg in the fully stretched position, but this has to be carefully done. Once the child has learned to feel the muscles' elastic limits, passive stretching is completely safe.

Most writers recommend warming up first, and then stretching, especially in relation to running.[99] The current author also feels that a warm shower or bath prior to stretching can serve the purpose of increasing the temperature and so preparing the muscles for stretching. In order to increase flexibility, stretching exercises should be repeated at the beginning and end of any exercise session, in both cases when the body has already been warmed up. However, if a muscle has been injured, or is specially tight for any reason, the passive stretching should be done prior to any other type of warming up. If this is not done, it is extremely easy for the child to over-stretch through not feeling the decreased elastic limit of the injured muscle. The passive stretching in this situation is preparation for further exercise. If the muscle group still feels tight despite careful stretching, it should not be stressed. Passive stretching should continue for as many days or weeks as it takes to make the muscle group normally pliable again. Passive stretching exercises should always be repeated after any exercise session, to prevent stiffness.

Muscle versatility

Mature adults of both sexes tend to be categorized into three main groups in terms of their favoured activity, which is usually the one they perform most easily and successfully. Some specialize in 'long endurance' activities of an aerobic nature, such as cycle-touring, marathons, triathlons, long swims and mountain or fell walking. Others are good at vigorous, short, mainly anaerobic activity, such as sprints, jumps and throws. The third group can do both, but neither to a high level. In other words, adults tend to be metabolic specialists. *Metabolism* refers to the predominant way in which a muscle produces its energy, either at a high rate for a short time, or at much lower rates for a longer time. The high and low rate systems dominate in 'fast' and 'slow' muscle respectively, and lead to exercise specialization. This specialization may be accompanied by a different basic body shape (technically called somatotype), which is genetically determined, together with the fibre profile of a person's muscle in terms of the percentage number of slow and fast muscle cells.

However, young children are much less specialized in this way. Below the age of about 10 for girls and 12 for boys, those who can run fast are usually the ones who can run far as well, although this gradually changes as they get older. While the muscle cell profiles are decided from birth, the patterns do not become fully effective until sometime between puberty and full maturity. Nevertheless, children may be directed towards specialization too soon. A survey of Little Athletic Clubs in Southern Australia concluded that specialization was starting too early, ignoring the fact that youthful competitors need particularly careful coaching according to their size, body proportions, lack of aerobic ability, level of neuro-muscular maturity and facility for skill acquisition.[100]

Body temperature control

The body gains heat from two sources, the metabolism occurring in its own cells, and the outside environment. All body cells, especially muscle, unavoidably convert 70 per cent of their chemical food energy into heat. During exercise the excess heat created could kill us, were it not dissipated by being radiated (like an electric fire) or convected (like a central heating panel) away, or by losing its energy through converting sweat into steam. Similarly, too great a loss of heat in a cold environment is countered by a very marked shutdown of skin bloodflow together with a rise in metabolic heat output through the repeated muscle contractions of shivering.

Children rely much more on radiation and convection to dissipate heat from the skin than adults. Because of this, and because they expend more chemical energy per kilogram of bodyweight than do adults, at high ambient temperatures it becomes progressively harder for them to dissipate heat from the skin. Adult men disperse about 70 per cent of their heat production by sweating, and most of the rest by convection and radiation. In trained Caucasian women, the figures are approximately 60–65 per cent and 40–35 per cent respectively, while in untrained women radiation and convection provide a greater percentage of their heat loss, with less lost through sweating. Children, like untrained women, are excellent radiators and convectors under normal conditions, losing approximately 50 per cent of their exercise heat load by these means, and 50 per cent through evaporation by sweating.

The sweating apparatus is developed by the age of 3, but only comes into full function around puberty. For instance, it has been noted that, in boys up to the age of 9 or 10, sweat rates are of the order of less than 350 ml per square metre of skin surface per hour, whereas by 12 to 13 this rises to between 400 and 500 ml, compared to an adult male's rate of 600 to 800 ml.[101] One litre of sweat evaporated from the skin can extract 580 calories of body heat. There are more sweat glands in a given area of a child's skin than an adult's, but they produce only one-third as much sweat per gland. Children tend to react like slim adults in whom the sweating mechanism has been artificially depressed. Children also tend to have higher skin temperatures.[102] The higher skin temperature hinders the flow of heat from body core to the periphery, because the heat gradient is less. The child's surface area provides an added reason for overheating problems if the environmental temperature is greater than the child's body temperature, or if the child is exposed to too much direct sun.[103]

Children have a high body surface-to-weight ratio. In general, for the same shape, the smaller an object is, the greater is its surface area relative to its mass. A young adult, 177 cm tall and weighing 64 kg, will have a skin surface area of 1.80 square metres. An 8-year-old, 128 cm tall and weighing 25 kg, will have a surface area of 0.95 square metres.[35c] Thus the young child has 36 per cent more skin surface for his weight. In too hot or too sunny an environment, that can lead to a faster rate of heating. Their high relative surface area, combined with their high exercising skin temperature, imply that, for a given heat transfer, children need a higher skin blood flow. Since children have a similar cardiac output for a given oxygen uptake and therefore for a given heat production, then the load on their circulation will be relatively greater, and a higher proportion of their cardiac output will be required for skin blood flow, leaving less to oxygenate muscle. Like adults, children are capable of acclimatization to heat, but they may take up to three times as long as adults to acclimatize fully.

Thus the endurance capacity of even highly trained athletic children is reduced compared to adults, through the limitations imposed on their cardiovascular systems by heat stress. The child's body has the added disadvantage of producing more heat per unit of bodyweight, partly due to the relative biomechanical inefficiency.

In too cold an environment, for example during swimming, especially outdoors in lochs or in the sea, the greater skin area of the child can lead to overcooling and hypothermia much sooner than in adults. Young children have less insulating fat beneath their skin compared to adults of both sexes.[104] Municipal and other pools in Britain are usually maintained at 25°C or above, but children may swim outdoors in temperatures of 20°C or much lower. This provides a potential risk, especially for the very keen, lean, small-sized swimmer, who may not be able to make up for the heat loss with the same powerful efforts as a competitive swimmer, for instance.[105] Euphoria, excitability, disorientation and reluctance to leave the water are warning signs of hypothermia in such situations. Obese children are at much less hypothermic risk in cold environments. Conversely, they are at greater risk in the heat: as they tend to sweat more than normal, they can be in greater danger of dehydrating.[106]

Thus, in summary, in many indoor and some summer outdoor sports situations, attention should be paid to frequent short rests (every twenty to thirty minutes), ideally with water available. Equally, care should always be taken with children exercising in the cold.

Dehydration

It is well known that many people who exercise at all levels of sport in hot environments do not drink enough to replace the fluid lost. If the rate of exertion is much above 70 per cent of maximum oxygen uptake, then the rate of absorption from the intestine may be unable to match the rate of sweat loss. However, at lower levels of exertion, dehydration can occur because people can simply fail to drink enough water, even when it is freely available.

With their ability to be active for long periods of time, and with their comparatively high breathing rates, children quite easily become relatively dehydrated. This may be exacerbated by the fact that, although the children become thirsty, they tend to drink only about two-thirds of what they lose.[107] Such dehydration will tend to happen on long hot days, or in warm sports halls or squash courts, and will be influenced by the length and total amount of the exercise, which, in squad or team training days or weekends, may be considerable. Voluntary dehydration is a recognized condition in some warmer countries, where it is known as 'thirst fever'. The 'fever' refers to the raised body temperature, but it is not, of course, due to any infection, being simply a combination of prolonged over-heating and too little fluid. It disappears as soon as the child is adequately rehydrated.

For endurance sport lasting longer than about an hour, a mixture of water, containing up to 0.3 g/litre of sodium chloride (salt), up to 0.28 g/litre of potassium chloride and up to 25 g/litre of sugar has been recommended as a useful liquid and electrolyte replacement drink.[35e] This takes into account the relatively low salt content of children's sweat. However, by far the main requirement is simply water, and children will tend to drink more of it if it is presented as orange squash, for example, especially with ice cubes, rather than plain water.

The child's view of exercise

There are various methods of rating a level of exertion in terms of its relative degree of hardship, and studies have been performed on children.[108] Exercise at equivalent levels is perceived as much easier by children than by adolescents, and hardest by adults.[109] Also, partly because of their greater emphasis on aerobic metabolism, their lower oxygen deficit and lower blood lactate levels, there is a much faster rate of recovery in young subjects. After a maximum oxygen intake test in the laboratory it may be several hours before adults can be persuaded into a further similar test. Yet many children want to repeat the test well within the hour, to see if they can do better!

Children's habitual higher rates of activity may result from their not perceiving it as particularly strenuous; adults may prefer their more sedentary style in part because they do perceive exercise as potentially fatiguing. The lesson for sport is that in strenuous work with youthful squads, the coach should call for short breaks with drinks every 20 minutes or so. This is to act as a check against dehydration, over-heating and simple exhaustion.

Conclusions

Children are not simply small adults. Indeed, they differ from adults qualitatively as well as quantitatively when it comes to exercise physiology. The wisest course seems to be to let children set their own levels of activity, yet that may amount to too little in many areas of Western society. In competition sport, on the other hand, there is some danger in activity levels being set too high. Problems arise when children are made to conform to adult concepts of sport, training and exercise, which is why the idea behind such excellent adaptations of sport as mini-rugby, short tennis, 'gym-Joey', racket-ball and soft-ball cricket should be extended into other activities.

The ability for endurance is present before puberty, but it has been suggested that it is not possible to recommend specialized prolonged endurance training as being beneficial for children, who naturally prefer to exercise in short, repeated bouts.[110] Many authorities consider that regular exercise before puberty increases the rate of development of physical abilities, including co-ordination and balance, and that it correlates significantly with strength, aerobic power and basic skills.[111] It is notable that individual differences in these attributes are strongly related to a lack of physical activity.[112]

It is important in childhood to train a wide variety of functions, such as aerobic and anaerobic endurance, strength, speed and co-ordination, by regular exercise. To concentrate too selectively on training only one attribute may be inappropriate and harmful during the first years of a sports career. It has been suggested that children have an excellent motivational feedback system and that when the training programme reaches above a level of tolerance, the child loses interest.[113] This feedback is overridden during growth, and

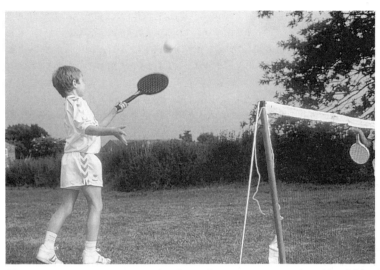

Short tennis: early training in eye–hand co-ordination, in a sport adapted for children.

during adolescence overloading becomes possible.

Thus a training programme for a child under 10 years old should be directed towards neuromuscular development and skills, and to a gradual, modest increase in aerobic and anaerobic power. Flexibility work, where appropriate, should be introduced between 10 and 12, and between 12 and 14 a successive increase in aerobic and anaerobic endurance and speed may be added. Strength and power training should follow sexual maturity and the resulting increased muscle mass.[114]

Whether at recreational, local league or elite level we should all try to ensure that physical activity in general, and sport in particular, does not become a form of child abuse, while recognizing its tremendous potential for allowing children to fulfil their development.

4 Children's Pains and Injuries

'Growing pains'

Young children may complain of a deep aching feeling in the thighs, behind the knees, or in the calves.[1] The pain can be severe, especially at the end of the day or during the night. Oddly, the legs are usually not sore to touch, and the muscles are not tight or in spasm. The problem can start when the child is very young, or in the early teens, and it can last for several years before disappearing. It may be worse after exercise, or when the child is tired. The leg pain often accompanies headaches and abdominal pain ('stomach ache'), so it is just possible that it is linked in some way to dietary allergies. Moving about or walking does not help the ache once it has started, but Aspirin might relieve it.

Growing pains usually affect both legs equally, and they may happen through the whole of the limbs, or just in one part. The exact cause of the pain is not known, although its pattern is well defined. There is no special treatment to cure growing pains, but as the problem disappears with time, you simply have to wait for nature to take its course. The child with growing pains can still do sport, but probably not intensively, if it seems that too much sport makes the symptoms worse.

'Clicking' joints

Many children have joints which make audible clicking or cracking noises during movements. Any joint can make this kind of sound, but it is usually more noticeable when the weight-bearing joints of the legs are affected. The clicks may come from just one joint, or from the same joint in each leg (for instance both ankles or both knees), or from several joints (for instance the feet, ankles, knees and hips on either or both legs). The sound may be more noticeable when the joint is moved after being held still, perhaps when the child first gets out of bed in the morning, or gets up from a chair.

The click might start following an injury, and it may be related to joint stiffness. More often, it has no obvious cause, and is probably simply a sign of relatively tight ligaments. Provided the click is not accompanied by pain, or linked to an obvious limitation of joint movement, there is no need to worry about it. If there is pain or limitation in the affected joint, the child should be checked by the doctor or orthopaedic specialist.

Children should not be encouraged to make their joints click by manipulating them. Some children enjoy making their finger joints crack by manipulating them, but this might cause later functional problems in the hands, so you should dissuade them.[2]

Clicking joints often stop being noisy as the child grows up. Sometimes exercising helps to make them quieter. There is certainly no need for a child to feel self-conscious about these joint sounds, although you should watch for any sign of pain or increased stiffness in the affected joints.

The need for diagnosis

Unfortunately, many children's pains are dismissed as 'simple growing pains' when in fact they are not. A child's pain should never be dismissed or ignored. Sometimes, you might feel that children should be discouraged from complaining of pain, partly so that they develop a 'stronger character', and partly because children's aches and pains tend to pass quickly. When a child does complain of pain, it can be tempting to treat it lightly, in case the child is exaggerating or making excuses to escape disliked activities. I feel it is better to err on the side of caution, and treat any complaint of pain seriously, until it is cured, either naturally, or through diagnosis and treatment. Even though one does not want to encourage a 'whingeing child syndrome', where the child invents a pain to attract adult attention or as an excuse, I feel it has to be recognized that although many aches and pains in childhood are trivial and pass without incident, a few can have serious consequences.

One young boy complained of pain in his right arm for a year, following an incident at the age of 10, when he threw a ball as hard as he could and experienced instant extreme pain. His parents encouraged him to exercise, in the hope that he would 'grow out of the problem'. When the pain became worse, the boy was seen by an orthopaedic specialist, who found a cyst in the arm bone (humerus). A bone graft was done, but the operation led to a sequence of problems which dominated most of the boy's teenage years. The parents were left regretfully wondering whether an earlier visit to the specialist would have saved their son some of the pain and disruption to his normal active life.

Some problems, tragically, may be so serious that there is little that can be done about them. A 15-year-old girl developed a gradual pain in the front of her right thigh. She enjoyed competitive rowing, and her family doctor felt that she must be suffering from an overuse strain in her quadriceps muscles, although the girl herself felt there was no cause for this. She had not been doing any unusual activities, nor had her rowing technique changed. She had not had any noticeable illnesses, either, although she had suffered the stress of her father's sudden death about a year previously. An only child, she had appeared to cope with the tragedy well, helping her mother to overcome her grief.

The girl was referred to a local hospital for physiotherapy, and was treated with ultrasound. Her pain became worse, so she was referred to a sports clinic through her rowing coach, with her doctor's approval. The doctor at the clinic immediately had her admitted to hospital, where tests showed that she had a massive malignant tumour in her thigh-bone (femur). Despite every effort by the doctors, and immense courage on the girl's part, she died some fifteen months later.

How widespread are children's injuries?

Fortunately, most children only suffer aches and pains through relatively simple injuries which can be diagnosed and treated successfully. As it is well recognized that the child is not simply a small-scale version of the adult, it follows that injuries affect the developing child's body differently, even though the stresses which produce injuries in adult and child may be similar. Like adults, children can suffer from overuse injuries, produced by repetitive stresses, and traumatic injuries, caused by obvious accidents such as a direct blow, fall or crush. Trauma can involve shearing, traction or compression forces, or a combination of these.

Children seem to recover quickly from accidental injuries, especially in the pre-teen years. By contrast, teenage overuse or misuse injury pains can linger for months. To complicate matters, children's problems sometimes develop without the child noticing any real pain to complain about. The child might limp, or stop using that part of the body, without being conscious why. As a responsible adult, you have to be observant, and notice any movement abnormality. You have to look for the cause if it cannot be resolved simply, so you may need to take the child to your doctor or sports clinic. Early diagnosis, followed by accurate treatment and rehabilitation exercises, can prevent minor problems from turning into major ones. In every case, full recovery is the priority.

Various studies have been done to describe and analyse the type and quantity of injuries affecting sporting children.[3–14] There is no doubt that children of all ages do get injured through sport, and that injuries occur both during supervised[11] and unsupervised sports.[13] Injuries can be specifically related to intensive sports practice,[15, 16] but they also happen during informal sports, physical education classes and play.

This author has treated injured children in general hospital practice, at the Crystal Palace National Sports Centre Injuries Unit, within elite sports squads, at major junior championships and in private practice. In the Crystal Palace Unit, which then operated free of charge, the majority of patients seen each year were children, and the majority of the children seen were aged 15–16.[17, 18] The pattern of children's injuries I treated in my private practice over some six years is illustrated in the table on p. 77.

Most of the surveys of children's injuries are based on patients presenting in clinics, surgeries or hospitals, so they reflect problems which have worried the child or responsible adults enough for professional help to be sought. There is little information about childhood aches and pains which have been ignored, or which have not been severe enough to need formal treatment, but which have been bad enough to be noticeable at the time, and remembered afterwards. However, clinical practitioners often feel that such background information can be important in assessing subsequent injuries. When assessing adult patients with musculoskeletal problems (relating to muscles, tendons, joints and bones), I always ask whether there have been any notable childhood injuries, aches or pains. During a six-year period in my private practice, for instance, it transpired that while the majority of adult patients could not recall whether or not they had suffered any significant childhood problems, 241 were positive that they had not, but 262 reported that they had: it seemed that many of these problems might have had a bearing on the patient's later problems.

Monitoring: the elite boys' squash squads

During five years working with the English junior boys' squash squads, I studied the patterns of injury, and advised the boys, their parents, coaches or teachers on injury treatment and prevention. The elite squads were the best players from around the country, who were selected for intensive training and coaching sessions, usually held over weekends. The players were divided into age-groups, ranging from under-10 to under-19. As part of the monitoring process, the players were questioned closely about their past and present injury patterns, besides being assessed biomechanically and physiologically. Very few of the 142 boys questioned and examined claimed to have had no injuries at all, although the majority of the injuries described did not require any kind of treatment other than a period off sport ranging from one day to two weeks. Some of the boys were seen only once, due to failure to regain selection to these elite groups, but most were seen several times during the five-year period. It was clear that the game carried a strong risk of specific injuries, particularly to the knee and the back, and that these were likely to begin at the earliest age when the player started to compete, and to persist or recur during the subsequent years.

Of the 734 injuries identified, 177 (24 per cent) were not directly caused by squash, although some of these injuries then interfered with squash playing. Football and running were the two main injury-causing sports apart from squash, although several injuries occurred through accidents unrelated to sport, such as car crashes and skylarking. The majority of the injuries were recognizably the result of playing squash. This was to be expected, as all the boys who earned selection for the weekend-long elite squad training sessions were inevitably highly motivated, competitive, and playing and training frequently and hard.

A typical case study showed that a very promising young player had a right-sided back injury at the age of 9, when he over-stretched for a ball; the problem lasted for several months. By 12, his left hip was turning in slightly, and both legs were relatively weak. He developed Osgood-Schlatter's 'disease' (p. 128) in the right knee, followed by knee-cap joint pain (p. 158) in the left knee, and continued to have knee pain playing squash until he was 14. When

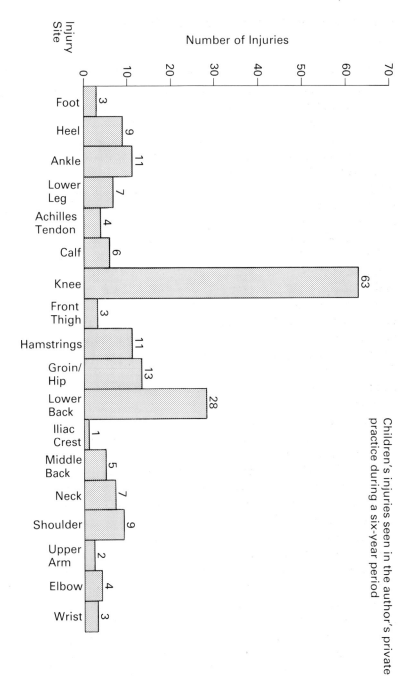

Children's injuries seen in the author's private practice during a six-year period

the boy and his parents were advised that he should rest from squash, or play less, or persevere with remedial exercises, they took little notice. The boy was very successful as he entered the senior game, unsurprisingly in view of the indomitable determination and courage which had helped him play through pain each season as a junior.

However, if top junior players start with injury cycles, their chances of escaping unscathed into the senior game and then into adult life beyond their squash-playing careers must seem remote. In October 1989, the professional squash players' journal, *Squash Proscene*, published a survey in which it was revealed that 92 per cent of the world's top thirty male players felt that they were likely to cause themselves permanent physical damage through playing the game at elite competitive level. Now that we know so much about injury causes and prevention, it is clear that a major task facing health professionals is persuading players, parents and coaches to accept our advice.

Possible after-effects and long-term risks of injuries

There have been scientific medical studies showing that there might be a link between sport, injuries and the development of degenerative joint disease (osteoarthritis). Ignoring injuries, and trying to play or run through pain can lead to long-term problems, including degenerative arthritis.[19] The danger of subsequent arthritis is worst when the injuries relate to the main weight-bearing joints of the leg, the ankle, knee and hip. As the knee is the joint most often injured through sport, there have been many studies of the long-term consequences, examining the changes in the knee's mechanics and protective mechanisms which injuries cause.[20, 21] Sports injuries, particularly those related to repetitive stress, are assumed to be important possible causes of hip and knee osteoarthritis.[22] There is a fear that these injuries in young people can lead not only to the later osteoarthritis which can happen to other people for a variety of different reasons, but also, in some cases, to unusually early degenerative problems. For instance, a major hip injury such as dislocation in a teenager can lead to subsequent painful osteoarthritis by the age of 21, if the injury is not treated efficiently and immediately.[23]

The injuries do not have to be major to cause later problems: for instance, it has been suggested that there might be a link between intensive athletic training, minor teenage hip deformity during growth development, and later degenerative disease (osteoarthritis) in the hip.[24] The unusual repetitive movements involved in sports can also cause early degenerative arthritis in non-weight-bearing joints in the trunk and arm: javelin throwing, for instance, can have this effect on the elbow, and it is feared that the new throwing technique required for the javelin since 1986 might also lead to early arthritis in the spine.[25] By contrast with the studies suggesting links between intensive sport, injuries and degenerative arthritis, it is also felt that 'reasonable exercise' using normal ranges of joint movement should not cause subsequent joint damage.[26]

How to deal with children's pains and injuries

Whenever a child complains of pain, or looks as though a movement or activity might be causing pain, you should stop him or her from doing sport, even if there has not been any obvious injury through the sport itself. The child may be able to tell you when the pain started, what caused it, and which movements make it worse. If not, you should try to glean as much information as you can, to pass on to the doctor. The child should be examined by the doctor as soon as possible: if the doctor cannot identify what is wrong, he may refer the child to a specialist for more detailed investigations in hospital.

Every adult involved in children's sport should be trained in first-aid procedures. Indeed, first-aid and emergency treatments should be learned by teenagers, preferably within their schooling, so that in any situation people know what to do accurately and quickly. Life-saving measures like artificial respiration (the 'kiss of life') and cardiac massage have to be instituted immediately in an accident where the victim's heart and breathing have stopped, especially as brain tissue deprived of oxygen is damaged much more quickly if the victim has been running about than if the accident happened at rest. You also have to know when not to move an accident victim, for instance if there is a risk that the spine is broken. For other broken bones and major wounds, you should know how to apply splints and dressings without causing further damage or producing infections.

More minor injuries are simpler to deal with: you can apply ice packs to a bruise, knock, sprain or strain, protecting the skin with a damp cloth or oil. Alternatively, you can simply rub ice cubes over the painful or swollen area. If no ice is available, cold water can be used, although it is a poor substitute. It has been suggested that ice packs containing crushed ice (not gel packs) should be applied directly to the skin, tied on with bandaging and left in place for up to thirty minutes.[77] This author usually applies ice for five to ten minutes in the first instance, according to how well the patient tolerates the cold.

You should never rub a muscle or joint immediately after it has been injured, as you can increase internal bleeding or fluid swelling, and in muscles you can even promote bone formation (technically called *myositis ossificans*). Applying heat in the form of a spray, lamp, hot water bottle or sauna in the immediate stages of an injury is also likely to congest the injury with excess fluid or blood. However, a warm (not hot) bath can help the body's overall circulation, indirectly helping the injury. If the victim can move the injured part without causing pain, gentle movements should be encouraged, and these may be more comfortable in a warm bath. Taking weight through an injured leg will probably make it more painful, so the patient should be given crutches, or carried off on a stretcher, chair, or between at least two people. The injured part should be elevated, so the patient should sit or lie with the foot up on a soft support. An injury to the arm should be protected in a sling.

For efficient first-aid, it is as important to know what *not* to do as what measures you should take. The best way to learn emergency techniques is to attend a first-aid course where you can practise resuscitation methods and bandaging. First-aid procedures are best kept simple, so that you do not try to do too much, or take on too much responsibility. Any major accident inevitably requires trained medical or paramedical help.[28, 29] You should always carry with you or have access to a basic first-aid kit, containing items like dressings, bandages or lengths of tubular bandaging, slings and a resuscitation airway. Schools, sports centres and clubs should have more extensive first-aid equipment readily available, such as stretchers, crutches and wheelchairs.

You should know where the first-aid equipment is kept, and where the nearest sources of ice and fresh water are. If children are playing on fields or pitches far from the nearest source, you should carry ice and clean water in jars. If any child in your care has a medical condition such as asthma or diabetes, you should make sure that the condition is properly controlled and that the child is taking any prescribed medicines correctly. You should ask the parents or medical officer what warning signs to watch for, and what you should do, in case the child gets into difficulties during exercise. If you are the parent of a child with a medical condition, it is your responsibility to make sure that any teacher, coach or other adult entrusted with your child is made aware of how to take proper care of him or her.

As an adult looking after a group of children, you should check whether all the children in your care have had anti-tetanus injections, so that you can pass the information on to the doctor, nurse or casualty officer, if any of them suffers a bad cut or graze. If a child has an open wound of any kind, he or she should not be allowed in the swimming pool or jacuzzi until it is completely healed, to prevent infections from entering the cut. Never allow children to eat while doing sport or running around. They should be specially discouraged from chewing gum, which might easily choke them if it gets trapped in the windpipe. You must know where the nearest telephone is, or carry a portable telephone, in case you need to call for an ambulance and emergency team.

When any accident happens, the child involved needs reassurance, and you will probably have to control and calm the other children around as well. It helps if you can ask them to do useful tasks, such as going for help, fetching water, or collecting up equipment. For a major accident the child has to be taken to hospital. Even for a seemingly more minor injury, it is prudent to have the child checked by a doctor, so that appropriate medical or rehabilitation treatment can be given, before the child tries to return to normal activities.

5 Why Do Children Get Injured?

- **Through doing the wrong sport**. Children should do sports they are capable of doing, at least to some level. The sport should be appropriate to the size and physical characteristics of the child. For instance, the young girl who is talented for gymnastics through courage and application, but is congenitally relatively inflexible, will probably be disappointed as well as injured if encouraged to aim at top competition honours where suppleness is a must. Children whose eye–hand co-ordination is poor cannot be expected to enjoy ball-handling or racket sports, or to play them efficiently. The child with flat feet or weak lower leg muscles is likely to jar the legs badly on trying to do gymnastics exercises involving jumping barefoot on a wooden floor.
- **Through doing the wrong type or amount of sport for the stage of development**. A very small child usually rides a small pony, and should not be put on a 16-hand showjumper which he or she could not sit on comfortably or control properly. The child's physical capacities change during and after the growth spurt: some activities are harder during this phase than in the pre-teen years. There are phases when the child's muscles become relatively tight, as bone length increases, and then relatively weak, so the child cannot keep up the same activity levels as previously.

As a child's size alters, the perspective of a court or pitch changes: for a small child a full-size football or rugby pitch is a vast area, and defending adult-sized goal posts is a major task. The very young child may be shorter than the tennis net, and may have to adjust playing technique radically on growing big enough to look over the net and to cover the court with fewer steps than previously. If a child has played mini-rugby or short tennis, the adult has to be careful to judge accurately when the child has grown enough to switch to the full-sized game.

• **Through too much sport.** This is a particular problem if the child likes one sport and wants to play it all day, every day. Constantly kicking a football about stresses the knees, while playing tennis or squash intensively pressurizes the arm, shoulder and back. On some synthetic surfaces, tennis players notice shin and knee soreness or pain, similar to a runner's aches and pains. Competitive swimming can stress the shoulders. The main problem is that each sport develops the growing body in a particular way, creating strong muscles in certain areas, and stiff or over-lax joints in other parts. Constant repetition of the same patterns of movement can lead to fatigue injuries in the muscles and tendons, or overload injuries in the joints; sudden unusual movements can over-stretch the body, causing wrenching or tears.

Over-training is especially dangerous in sports involving a limited range of repetitive movements, like rowing or running. The child may show signs of struggling: for instance in running, if the thigh muscles are not strong enough to keep the correct pattern of

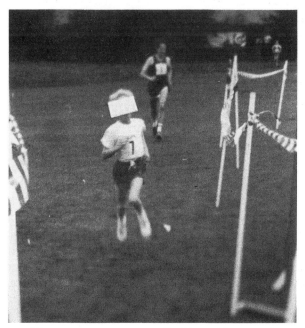

When a young runner goes too far, hips and knees turn in.

movements going, the hips and knees tend to turn in, throwing the feet outwards. The combination of excessive training plus inefficient body movements places damaging stresses on the major weight-bearing joints, especially the hips. An important antidote is to make sure that the child varies his or her activities, and does not do the same sport every day.

• **Through using the wrong size of equipment.** An adult-sized tennis racket places a great strain on a child's arm, creating inappropriate leverage, and over-development of the arm, shoulder and trunk muscles on one side to cope with the load. Children should learn racket sports, throwing events and any ball game with equipment appropriate to the size of the child. They should not change to adult-sized equipment until their growth and development justify it – the change should not be made on the basis of age. The worst reason for choosing a particular racket or other equipment is on the basis that 'my friends have it and like it'. Sports equipment should be chosen on a personal basis, objectively. The coach should teach the parent or older child how to choose suitable equipment.

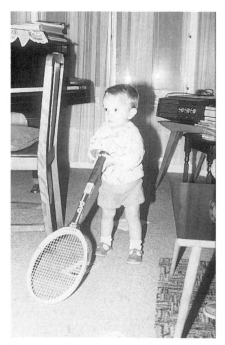

Equipment should be size-matched to the child.

Cycle racing is a sport where fine adjustments can make the difference between efficient pedalling and damaging shearing stresses, especially on the knees and back. Young cyclists have to keep checking that their bicycles are properly adjusted for their increasing height, and they will need to change bicycle frames as they out-grow them. Children who have a bicycle for fun or transport must take care to keep the saddle as high as possible, to avoid abnormal stresses on the knee-cap joint. For the same reason, they should stand up in the pedals when they cycle up hills.

• **Through lack of appropriate protective equipment**. Many sports require protective clothing or shields: if the parent cannot afford to kit the child out properly, the child should not participate in that sport. The armour needed for tae kwon do or the padded clothing vital for ice hockey, American football or fencing are very expensive. You may be reluctant to invest in this for a growing child who will certainly grow out of the gear, and may also grow out of the enthusiasm for the sport. Some clubs operate a hire system for special equipment of this kind. Otherwise, the child could be restricted to learning techniques only, without being allowed into contact situations, until old enough to take some responsibility for the investment.

The very young child has a soft skull, so any child learning to ski before the age of 7, for instance, should wear a helmet. Helmets are important at any age for sports like skateboarding, horse-riding, American football or cycling. The boxer's helmet has to protect the ears as well as the head. For many sports, including lacrosse and hockey, the helmet needs an integral face-mask. Fencing is a sport which requires a face-mask but not a helmet. Water polo players use a protective cap which protects their ears from trauma. Gum shields fitted by a dentist should be used for sports like rugby and boxing. Goggles protect the eyes from infection or irritation through swimming in chlorinated water. Ear defenders are vital for the older child who practises clay pigeon shooting. Special thick belts should be used to protect the back during motorbike scrambling and weightlifting. 'Boxes' to protect the genitals are needed for boys in sports like cricket, boxing, or for the goalkeeper in field hockey. Elbow and knee protectors are widely used for skateboarding, but many types are inadequate: parents and children have to learn to judge which sports accessories are fashion items only, and choose protectors which provide proper cover and shock absorption. Shin guards are

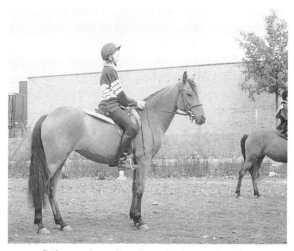

Riders need a well-cushioned helmet or hard hat.

essential for sports like football and field hockey.

All protective equipment should fit the child, and should be worn securely fastened in place. It should be replaced as the child grows out of it, or at the first signs of wear which might reduce its effectiveness.

• **Through inadequate skill training**. Every sport requires some level of skill, and the child, like the adult, should learn how to perform the movements of the sport efficiently. Technique is a complex problem in sports involving high skill levels, like tennis and golf. Tennis illustrates how there is no such thing as an absolute model for technique: top players use a variety of styles, some one-handed, others two-handed on both forehand and backhand, some two-handed for the backhand only. No particular style guarantees victory against the others. The game's technique has evolved partly through individual innovations, and partly because of the development of new materials for rackets, balls and court surfaces. The mistake is for learners to imitate styles which they cannot achieve, because they lack the strength, flexibility or timing.

The good coach or teacher shows children the basic methods involved in a sports technique, and then elaborates on it in relation to the children's individual abilities. Sports technique requires constant adaptation: the child grows, or new variations and refinements are introduced by top exponents of the particular sport, which can then be assimilated by junior players and adapted within their own capabilities.

• **Through inappropriate fitness training.** Introducing formal fitness training too early as a background for sports is likely to cause problems if the child is not physically or mentally mature enough for it. Fitness training requires an understanding of its aims: for instance stretching exercises should only be done within the muscles' elastic limits, and strength training should not over-stress the body. The very young child may not understand these limits, nor the progressive nature of training.

Doing the wrong type of fitness training in relation to the child's sport is another mistake. The teenager in a competitive sport inevitably gets involved with fitness training, and the programme has to be devised as a relevant background, including protective exercises. For instance, rowing requires strength and muscle endurance in the legs, trunk, shoulders and arms, so a weight-training programme should be geared to all these areas. The sport stresses the back, making rowers relatively round-shouldered, so protective exercises should include back extension movements, for instance lying on the stomach and lifting the trunk and legs backwards. Canoeing, on the other hand, depends mainly on upper body and arm strength. Therefore running is not the right type of aerobic training exercise specifically for canoeing, but, together with weight-training for the legs, it is useful as background work to improve the canoeist's body balance.

Overdoing fitness training leads to injuries through fatigue, and sometimes through faulty technique, especially in weight-training. The squash player who does too much distance running for training is likely to be slowed down on court, and put at risk of suffering the overuse injuries associated with running but not with squash, especially stress fractures in the leg bones.

• **Through insufficient preparation.** Like adults, children should start any new sport gradually, learning techniques bit by bit, practising them on a limited scale at first, and gradually building up the amount they play. Sessions should be spaced out, at least at first, to allow the body time to adjust and recover.

The warm-up is an important preparation for any exercise session, and the warm-down helps prevent stiffness following a workout. Like fitness training, the warm-up and warm-down are disciplines for older children (teenagers) who can understand what they are doing and why.

● **Through inadequate supervision**. Young children, especially, have no sense of potential danger, so, left to themselves, they can take unnecessary risks. Games of 'dare' running across railway lines or busy roads are examples. Equally, they can expose themselves to risk inadvertently, for instance by failing to notice a car coming because they are intent on chasing a ball. In a weights gym, unsupervised children inevitably try to lift the heaviest possible loads. As children cannot assess safety factors, they may try out dangerous moves on gymnastics equipment or trampolines. They may not notice when crash mats are not in place. They may try to dive into shallow water, or swim too far in one go for their strength.

Uncontrolled children not only put themselves at risk, but they can create dangers for those around them. They do not necessarily take account of other people when they are running or cycling around. They may be concentrating on throwing a javelin or discus, and fail to notice people moving into their throwing area. Lack of

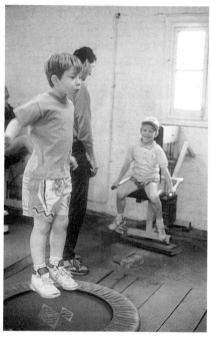

Children exercising under supervision in the author's gym.

awareness of other people is especially dangerous when everyone is moving at speed, as in surfing, downhill skiing or tobogganing. Children can sometimes be dangerously rough with each other, for instance when imitating fights they may have seen on television.

• **Through poor discipline.** Children respond to discipline, and often create their own discipline in organizing games among themselves with appropriate rules. However, it is also true that children can lapse very quickly into indiscipline: when a teacher leaves a classroom in any school, there is likely to be hubbub, even pandemonium, as the children celebrate their release from control. Children like to test how far they can go before they are brought into check by an adult. In team games and many individual sports, safety often depends on the discipline of the players, and this in turn depends on the strict application of the rules. In squash, for instance, players have to learn straight away that play must stop if there is any danger to either player. Equally, the marker or referee may have to apply the rules to prevent rough or intimidating play. In rugby, it is against the rules, and extremely dangerous, to collapse a scrum. The physical education teacher, coach or referee has to keep full control of all the players in order to ensure that they know and obey the rules.

• **Through inappropriate size-matching.** In team sports involving confrontation and tackling, such as rugby, football (soccer) and American football, relatively under-developed children should not be matched against those who are more mature physically. Individual combat sports like judo, wrestling and boxing are generally weight-matched to provide fair and safe contests.

• **Through an unsafe environment.** Children are usually not aware of potential dangers in the sports hall, swimming or diving pool, gymnasium, court or pitch. The responsible adult has to make sure that there are no protruding objects or obstacles in the children's way; that floors are not slippery or wet; that crash mats are securely in place if children are jumping down from apparatus to the floor; that mats cover the floor space properly for sports like judo; that goal posts for rugby or American football are padded; and that floor and ground surfaces are free from dirt, stones or sharp objects. It is equally important for children not to wear clothing with protruding buckles, or jewellery such as rings, earrings, bracelets or neck chains during sport.

The ambient temperature is an important consideration. If it is very hot, children must be encouraged to drink plenty of water, to prevent cramps and dehydration. They should wear sun hats if they are standing outside for long periods, for instance in cricket matches. Clothing should be light, preferably of natural materials like cotton to help sweat evaporation. Children should learn from an early age to put on a sweatshirt or jumper when they finish hard exercise, and, more importantly, to take a shower or bath and change their clothes.

If it is very cold, children must be properly dressed to prevent chills. Extreme cold can damage the growing epiphyses (bone ends), especially in the hands, so children should not be allowed to play in the snow without gloves, nor should they stay outdoors in the cold for long periods at a time. For watersports in relatively cold climates, children should use wetsuits. They should not be allowed to swim in cold water for any length of time, because of the risk of hypothermia. In any cold environment, children should keep warm by moving about: they should not be allowed to sit still and then go into action without warming up, for instance when substituting in a football match. Children should wear tracksuits if the weather is cold, and keep the tracksuit on until warm enough to discard it without discomfort. The tracksuit should be put on again immediately after the end of the activity.

• **Through poor shoes**. If shoes do not fit properly, they can compress the joints in the mid- and forefoot, causing bunion-like distortions. Toe-nails can be chafed and torn off, possibly with long-term damage to the nail-bed. Compression of the foot joints can have a 'knock-on' effect to the lower leg and knee. If sports shoes provide the wrong support for the foot joints, or too little support, the whole leg may be affected, mechanically, up to the hip. For this reason, sports shoes should be flexible rather than rigid, allowing the small foot joints complete freedom of movement.

Sports shoes should not be used for everyday wear, and then for sports as well, if at all possible. The synthetic materials of modern shoes make the feet swell if they are worn for long periods. The shoes are also too soft, and do not provide enough support for the repetitive pressure of walking, especially under the heel. Constant usage wears out sports shoes very quickly, and they lose their shock-absorbing or supportive qualities sooner than they show external signs of wear and tear. Modern sports shoes can deteriorate just with time, even without being worn, so a pair that has been held in stock for a year or two may not be a bargain, even at a reduced price.

Children should learn to look after their shoes: they should be discouraged from taking them off without untying the laces, as this stretches the shoes and makes the sides collapse. Velcro fastenings may be more suitable for the young child. Sports shoes should be kept clean, and allowed to dry out thoroughly if they become wet. They should not be kept in a bag for long after being worn. They should be checked frequently, so that the insoles or outer soles can be replaced immediately, when necessary.

Many sports require special shoes. Field hockey needs soccer-style boots when played on grass, but specially adapted trainers when played on synthetic surfaces. Tennis players need smooth-soled shoes for soft indoor carpet surfaces, but more robust gripping soles for the very hard synthetic surfaces, and a lighter shoe for dry grass or clay courts. For court games, the child should learn to test the friction characteristics of sports shoes, in order to wear the right shoes for the surface. Wearing the shoe, the player draws the sole across the surface: if the shoe judders, the grip is too harsh; if the shoe slides, there is not enough grip. While cross-country or longer distance runners need fairly thick, cushioned soles, tennis, squash and badminton players need thinner soled shoes, so that they can feel the floor under their feet in order to twist and pivot efficiently. Flared soles are not suitable for most sports, as they make the foot unstable.

Insoles often wear out more quickly than the outer parts of the shoe, and this can create blister problems, besides altering the foot and leg mechanics. Cushioned insoles or heel supports are often needed to protect the child from the jarring stresses of running or jumping. The life of a shoe can be extended, in many cases, if worn insoles are replaced with better materials for shock absorption. The child with very flat or weak feet may need specially made insoles, called orthotics, to correct the foot mechanics. Orthotics are fitted by a podiatrist or chiropodist, or sometimes by a physiotherapist or occupational therapist. The growing child should be re-assessed at frequent intervals to check whether new corrective insoles are needed.

Friction from sports shoes causes not only blisters, but also deeper damage. A badly shaped heel counter can cause a hardened lump on the back of the heel, commonly called a 'pump bump'. Raised backs (heel tabs) to the shoes, or boot seams which rub can make the Achilles tendons sore and thickened.

Shoes should be foot-shaped and the right fit. Sports shoes should not fit snugly to the feet, as there is always a certain amount of swelling when the feet get hot during activity. Parents who choose slightly bigger sizes to allow room for growth have to allow a little extra for this when buying sports shoes for their children. Children may need several pairs of sports shoes if they do different sports. Replacing them when necessary is expensive, but it can save a lot of problems in the child's feet and legs.

• **Through playing when injured, or not fully recovered from injury.** Even a minor injury inhibits normal movement in the injured area, making the child compensate. For example, the slightest limp throws stresses onto the joints above or below a leg injury, while an elbow injury can cause secondary stresses down to the hand or up to the shoulder. If the child tries to continue sport, playing through an injury, further strains are likely to result. This is why it is so important for children to receive accurate rehabilitation guidance for their injuries: full recovery is not just the absence of pain, but full strength, stretch and co-ordination in the injured part.

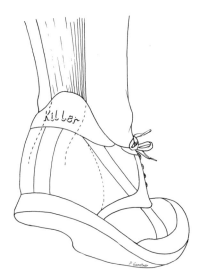

A high shoe back puts pressure on the Achilles tendon

• **Through playing when over-tired or ill.** Children rarely know their own limits, and they often fail to realize when they are too tired to keep up their activities safely. Paradoxically, it is when a child is almost exhausted that he or she is likely to be most stubborn about continuing a favourite pastime. Accidents can happen easily in this situation, as the child may become unco-ordinated and fall, or lose control of equipment. Excessive fatigue can also be linked to illnesses or infections, so you have to keep careful control, and not allow or encourage the child to continue a game or sport in the face of obvious signs of tiredness or poor health. Sometimes virus infections can cause muscle or joint pain that seems just like the pain of an injury, especially around the shoulder blades, upper back and rib cage. It is important to make the child rest, in bed if necessary, for as many days as are needed to let the fatigue or illness pass completely. The child should not be allowed to continue sport just because antibiotics have suppressed the symptoms of the illness. Any associated pains will ease off as the child's health recovers. The adult often has to apply strong discipline to prevent the child from returning to sport too soon in this situation.

6 Injury Prevention

If you are aware of the possible causes of children's injuries, you can avoid the preventable problems by anticipating potential dangers and taking necessary action against them. Many injuries can be avoided simply through the common sense and watchfulness of the responsible adult. To protect children from doing the wrong sport in relation to their stage of development, you can judge 'by eye' if the child seems to be struggling unduly to keep up, or if a piece of equipment looks too heavy or unwieldy for the child. However, the most difficult aspect of injury prevention is recognizing when the child's body development is changing in such a way as to alter the child's capacity for physical effort and exercise. It is one of the paradoxes of children's sport that at some phases of development the child can achieve more, physically, than at a slightly later phase, even though the child is older and more mature. You need to be aware of this danger, in order to predict when it is likely to happen, and to recognize when it actually is happening.

The growth spurt is an important landmark in a child's physical development. Increased leg length is often the most noticeable sign of a surge in growth: the child might suddenly look long-limbed and gangling, because the increase in bone length has stretched out the muscles, making them look somewhat thin. Bone growth inevitably involves a phase where the attached muscles are relatively weak and tight: the child may not be able to touch his or her toes any more, standing up, or may feel unusually tired during normal sport. Once the growth spurt has passed, the child fills out, and there may be a period of suddenly increased strength, especially in boys. This may be accentuated by sports involving heavy loading, especially power-lifting or throwing events. Heavy work, such as jobs on a farm or in a

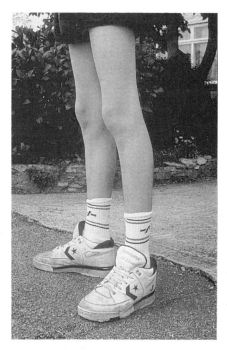

*Limb growth in a 15-year-old boy, showing tight hamstrings
and poorly developed quadriceps muscles.*

dairy, can also contribute to the development of a heavily muscled
build in a strongly built teenager. However, a strong muscular
development is often accompanied by decreased flexibility, as muscles are at their strongest in their middle range of work, when they
are not fully stretched out. If muscles gain bulk and strength without
being stretched to their full length they become tight and shortened,
and the teenager may be described as 'muscle-bound'.

As the child's structural development does not happen as a
smooth continuous process, it is vital to avoid the mistake of planning
sports participation on the basis of a continuing progressive plan.
The most efficient way to judge the child's physical capacity for sport
is through tests and measurements to assess the various relevant
parameters. Some types of testing are complicated, involving sophisticated, expensive equipment such as the muscle measuring
machines like the Kin Com, Lido or Cybex. Most of these machines
are built for adult use, so they are only used for older teenagers and

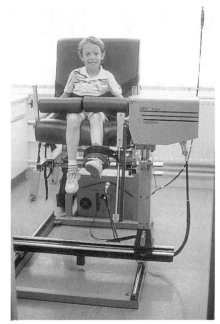

Muscle testing on the Lido, an adult-sized machine.

are not adapted for young children. However, many useful tests can be done 'in the field', using simple methods which still provide reasonably accurate and very useful information.

Monitoring and measurements

In most countries, babies are monitored to ensure that they are growing up in a normal way. At school, checks on development and health screening may be performed by the medical officer, school nurse or physiotherapist, or sometimes by the physical education teachers. If a child has development problems, more detailed checks and investigations may be carried out at a hospital or clinic.[1]

Early monitoring is used as a method of identifying potentially serious problems in children, but it could also be used more widely for fitness and health assessment. Physiological testing is used for adults not only to find early signs of heart disease, but also to assess their fitness, with a view to improving it. It has been recognized that the tests used for adult physiological measurements are not necessarily valid for children.[2] The Council of Europe has promoted a simple battery of tests for assessing schoolchildren's fitness, partly in order to gather information, and partly as a means of encouraging children to be aware of their physical well-being and its dependence on physical activity.[3]

Fitness monitoring has been more widely used for children involved in competitive sport than for those who are relatively inactive or not particularly talented. In the United States, for instance, monitoring competitive athletes and sports players is an important part of their background preparation. The emphasis is placed on monitoring in order to identify problems which can be corrected, and those which mean that the athlete should not participate in competitive sport(s). Very detailed monitoring procedures for high-school, college, elite and professional competitors have been laid down, partly for legal reasons, so that there are accurate records in case of any litigation involving the athlete, and partly in order to correct the athlete's weaknesses, and therefore improve performance.[4–11] It has also been suggested that increased competitiveness in children's sport has led to increased injuries, and that evaluation of the child's musculoskeletal system can help injury prevention.[12] The pre-season or 'pre-participation' assessment is usually only done on an annual basis. The evaluation is primarily geared towards serious competition, whatever the age-group of the athletes under test.

In Britain, thorough testing is generally only available to children involved in a particular sport, even though part of the testing might aim to establish the child's suitability for that or some other sport. The governing body of each sport usually organizes and pays for the testing process, which might be done 'in the field' or in a laboratory. For instance, the junior boys' elite squash squads were usually tested by a visiting physiologist and physiotherapist at their weekend training venues round the country, whereas the girls attended a motor performance laboratory. A special monitoring project, called the Training of Young Athletes project (TOYA) was launched in Britain in 1987. Funded by the Sports Council, and carried out by the Institute of Child Health, it set out to determine the effects of prolonged training and competition on youngsters' development, studying competitors in gymnastics, swimming, football and tennis. By 1989, preliminary results from the study were being presented and discussed.[13–17]

Regular monitoring of the sporting child serves three main

purposes. Firstly, medical and/or injury problems are revealed, so they can be treated early, or avoided if they are still in an incipient phase. Secondly, the child's state of development and physical capabilities are objectively assessed, so suitable levels and types of physical activity can be prescribed. The results of training or playing programmes can be measured, and the programmes modified accordingly. This can help prevent over-training and its related problems of injuries and staleness. Thirdly, the records of these assessments can provide objective data about the relationships between sports activities, growth, and medical and physical problems arising during the growth years.

The more scientific information we accumulate in this way about children in sport, the more we can turn *suggestions* on avoiding problems into *certainties* and confident advice. Children who participate in this process gain benefit for themselves, and for future generations who will be given advice on injury prevention, health promotion and performance improvements on the basis of an increasingly broad range of information.

This author believes that monitoring should be ongoing, and preferably carried out at least twice a year, or more often if this is practicable. The child or teenager involved in competitive sport may be monitored by the coach, exercise physiologist, physiotherapist, athletic trainer or doctor. One or several people may be involved in the monitoring process, and the results should be made known to all the people responsible for the child's general welfare and sporting career, as well as to the child. Repeat tests are usually more accurate if they are always carried out by the same person. The checks can be done at the sports centre, club or school where the sporting activity takes place, or in a special laboratory equipped with sophisticated equipment.

Some of the detailed monitoring procedures applied to talented sporting children could be part of a more general process of evaluating children's growth and health, even when they are not involved in competitive sport. For the normally active child, monitoring physical capacities is useful for assessing postural development and general fitness. Monitoring can also reveal factors which might lead to later problems like osteoarthritis, so preventive measures can be instituted. The evaluation can be used to make the child more aware of health matters such as the importance of diet, dental care and exercise, with obvious long-term benefits.

While some aspects of fitness monitoring depend on specialists, such as doctors, physiologists, physiotherapists and psychologists, many checks can easily be carried out by parents and coaches. The simplest records you can keep of a child's growth are changes in height, weight and shoe size, which can be noted at intervals of one, three or six months. A useful record is to take the child's pulse reading first thing in the morning: the teenager should learn to take his or her own pulse. If you take a reading of this *basal pulse* regularly for a couple of weeks, you will establish what it should be on average (allowing for the fact that it may seem to fluctuate a lot, according to different factors like excitement or fatigue). The basal pulse is a useful guideline: if it is raised by ten beats or more above the normal rate, *and the child is feeling under the weather or slightly unwell,* he or she should not do strenuous exercise that day, as it may be the first sign of an infection. It is also useful to keep a clean thermometer in the house to take the child's temperature if there are signs of illness, as a raised temperature is a definite bar to sport or exercise of any kind.

You can also do the physical tests such as those listed below. The easiest way to learn how to take reasonably accurate measurements is to be shown how by a physiotherapist. Although the tests *can* be done on very young children, they are more appropriate for older children and teenagers who can co-operate and follow instructions, and who may be interested in the reasons for the tests and the significance of the results.

With these tests, you are aiming to assess how good the child's co-ordination is, how strong the child's different muscle groups are, how flexible the muscles are, and whether there are obvious areas of weakness, tightness or body imbalance. There is no absolute standard for the child to match up to, but any specific weaknesses identified should be corrected by remedial exercises set out by the physiotherapist, so that on re-testing they are improved or corrected. The test exercises themselves can double as remedial exercises. A more comprehensive selection of therapeutic and protective exercises for stretching, mobilizing and strengthening each part of the body is given in the author's previous book, *Sports Injuries, a Self-Help Guide.*[18]

The record you keep of the tests should start with details of the time and date of the test, when the child last ate a meal, whether the child has drunk enough water, whether he or she has been ill at all during the previous two weeks, and whether he or she feels particularly tired (for instance because of doing examinations). The tests are best done barefoot, but if the child has to wear shoes for some reason such as skin infections, you should record this as well. Clothing should be light: although it is easier to judge body movements with the child undressed down to underwear, many children and teenagers are shy, so they should be allowed to wear a light tee-shirt and shorts, as for normal sports.

Most children enjoy both the attention and the challenge involved in physical testing. However, if a child shows any sign of physical or emotional distress during the tests, he or she should be allowed to stop straight away, as there is nothing to be gained by forcing a child to do the movements unwillingly or in fear. If the child seems to be suffering physically, you should take a pulse reading: if the pulse is racing, it may be the first sign of an infection like a cold or 'flu, so the child may need to rest, and perhaps see the family doctor.

Basic biomechanical tests (and remedial exercises)

1. **Balance**: the child stands on one leg, barefoot, as still as possible for as long as possible. The test is done on each leg in turn, and you time the child until the balance is lost. If the child can manage two minutes without wobbling, the test is repeated, but with eyes closed. For children with excellent balance, these tests can also be done on the wobble board (p. 136).

2. **Toe control**: the child presses his or her toes flat down onto the floor, not letting them curl. In the second part of the test, the child lifts the outer four toes off the floor slightly, and tries to press the big toe down flat, on its own. These tests are done barefoot, one foot at a time. A record is made of the ease or difficulty with which the child achieves the movements, and any noticeable difference between each foot. A better record is kept if you have a weighing scale, and position the child with the toe tips on it, to measure the amount of pressure the child can exert using only the toes.

3. **Foot–leg**: the child balances on the balls of the feet, and walks on the toes, taking ten steps forwards, backwards, then sideways in each direction; then ten steps are done walking on the outer edges of the feet in all directions; then on the inner edges of the feet, and finally on the heels. The movements are done barefoot on grass or a carpet, and any difficulty or imbalance between the feet is noted.

4. **Calf muscle function**: the child stands on one leg, barefoot on a firm surface, and goes up and down on the toes of that leg, keeping the knee straight. You count the number of movements achieved on each leg, and note any difficulty, such as inability to keep the knees straight. To test muscle endurance, you can count the repetitions achieved while timing the child over thirty seconds or one minute, according to the size of the child, or whether he or she looks over-fatigued in a short space of time.

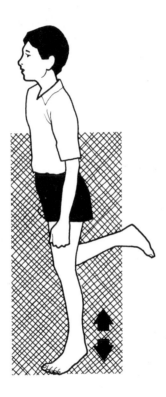

5. **Calf flexibility**: the child stands with one leg in front of the other, and bends the forward knee, keeping the hind foot flat on the floor and the hind knee straight, until the calf is fully stretched. You take the perpendicular measurement from the tibial tubercle just below the knee, and note how far behind or in front of the toes the tape lies (see illustration on next page).

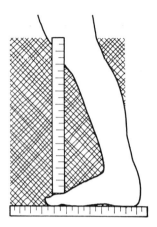

6. **Leg co-ordination**: the child stands on one leg, bends that knee keeping the foot flat on the floor, then straightens the leg to go up on the toes, lowers the foot flat to the floor and then bends the

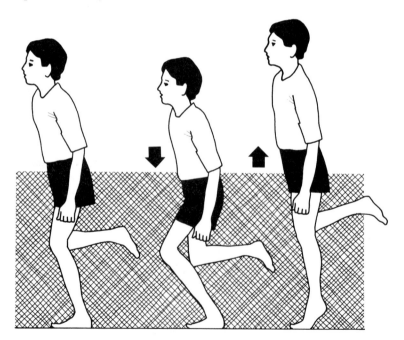

knee to start the movement again. The test is done barefoot, and you count the number of continuous movements the child achieves on one leg without losing balance, then repeat on the other leg.

7. **Knee, vastus medialis function**: the child sits on the floor with straight legs. You stabilize one thigh by pressing it down, and straighten the knee on that side fully, passively, by pulling the heel upwards towards the ceiling. You then ask the child: 'Straighten your knee as hard as you can, keeping your toes pointing up to the sky.' When the thigh muscles are tightened, you let go of the heel. Having measured the initial degree of passive (hyper)extension with a vertical ruler alongside the foot, you measure the amount that the heel drops when you let go of the foot. For the child whose knee(s) cannot straighten fully passively, the test is done with the knee supported on a measured block. (The test is done on each knee.)

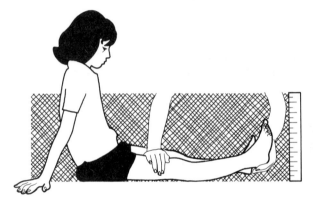

8. **Quadriceps flexibility**: the child lies prone (on the stomach), bends one knee, and you push that heel gently towards the seat, noting if the heel touches the seat, or measuring how far from the buttock muscle the heel reaches.

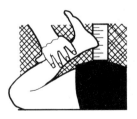

9. **Knee function**: the child stands straight, with legs slightly apart, goes up on the toes and then bends the knees to go down slowly into the squat position, keeping the back as straight as possible. You note any difficulty, or differences between the two knees.

10. **Hamstring efficiency**: the child lies prone and bends one knee, kicking his or her heel towards the seat. Timing the child over thirty seconds or one minute, you count the repetitions in which the child strikes the floor then the seat on one leg, then repeat the exercise on the other leg. If the child cannot touch the seat with the heel, you place a 'filling', such as books or thicknesses of wood, so that the heel just strikes it, and count the repetitions in the same way.

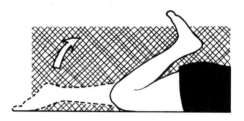

11. **Hamstring flexibility**: the child sits on the floor with legs straight, and reaches forwards, keeping the toes pointing up, and back and knees straight. You note whether the child can reach beyond his or her toes, and measure the distance between the big toe and the middle finger on each side.

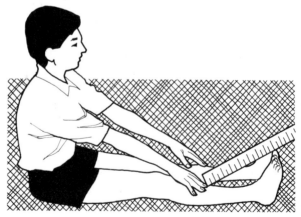

12. **Squat-and-reach endurance**: the child stands about a foot away from a wall, and squats down to touch the floor, then stands, going up on the toes to stretch up as far as possible to touch the wall above his or her head, while you mark the point reached on the wall. Then, timing over thirty seconds or one minute, you count the number of times the child can achieve the same movements of touching the floor and stretching up to the marker on the wall.

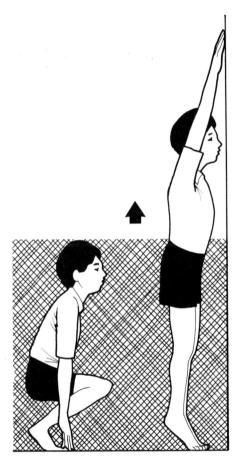

13. **Hip splay**: the child lies down with legs relaxed so that the feet and legs roll outwards. You can judge by eye whether one foot splays out more than the other, and if so whether the knee on that side is also turned out to the same degree. Otherwise, you can

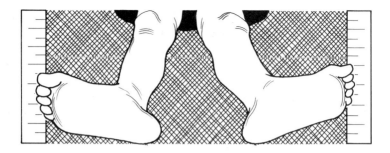

measure the vertical distance from the tip of the little toe to the ground on each side.

14. **Hip and pelvis**: the child stands on one leg, hitches the other vertically upwards towards the waist, leaning slightly towards that leg, then lifts the free leg straight out sideways, and slowly lowers it again. The test is done on each side, and any difficulty or imbalance is noted. (Inability to hold the pelvis level when standing on one leg is

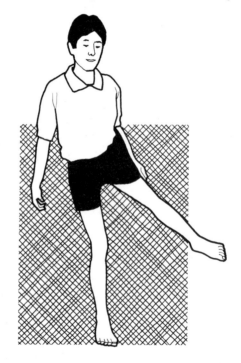

called 'Trendelenburg's sign': the unsupported leg tends to drop downwards from the hip through abductor muscle weakness.)

15. **Hip joint mobility**: the child lies supine (on the back) with legs straight. You gently lift one of the child's legs, bend it at the hip and knee, and press the knee towards the chest and from side to side, in an arc inwards and outwards. You note any discomfort the child feels at any part of the movement, and any lack of smoothness as you guide the knee from side to side.

16. **Hip adductor flexibility**: the child sits on the floor with knees bent, and soles of the feet together at a comfortable distance in front of the body. The legs are relaxed to allow the knees to fall sideways. You can measure the vertical distance from the floor to the knee on each side, or you can note by eye any difference between the two sides.

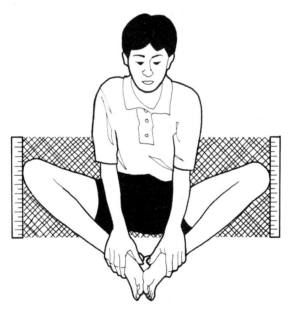

17. **Hip and lumbar extension flexibility**: the child lies prone (on the stomach) and pushes up on the hands as far as possible, straightening the elbows, lifting the upper trunk and stretching the head back, but keeping the hips in contact with the floor. You measure the vertical distance between the floor and the chin, then the floor and the top of the breast-bone (technically the *sternal notch*).

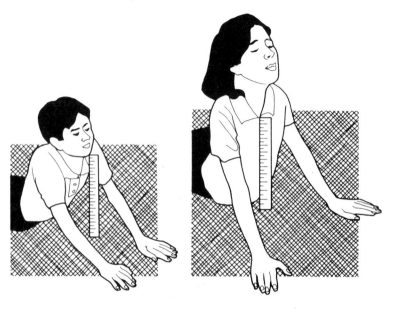

18. **Hip and side-trunk**: the child lies on one side, resting on the elbow, with trunk and legs straight, and looking straight ahead. Balancing on the elbow and foot, the child lifts the hips up sideways as high as possible, then slowly lowers. The movement is repeated three to five times. The test is done on either side, and the height of the hip lift can be measured, or judged by eye. Any difficulty or difference between the two sides is noted. You can also test the muscle endurance by counting how many movements the child can achieve in thirty seconds or one minute first on one side, then the other.

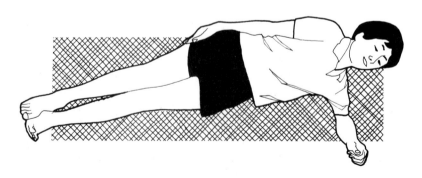

19. **Trunk sideways mobility**: the child stands upright with his or her back against a wall, and bends sideways as far as possible, keeping the back and head just in contact with the wall. You measure the distance between the tip of the middle finger and the side of the knee.

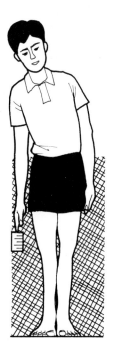

20. **Pelvis and trunk**: the child lies on his or her back with knees bent, feet flat on the floor, and sits up to touch the hands to the knees, keeping elbows straight and feet down on the floor. If the child cannot achieve the movement, you record this, but if it is easy, the test is done with arms crossed to place the hands on opposite shoulders, and the child tries to bring the elbows up to the knees. If this is difficult, you note it. You can assess muscle endurance by counting the number of sit-ups the child can achieve in thirty seconds or one minute, using the easier or harder version of the bent-knee sit-up according to the child's ability.

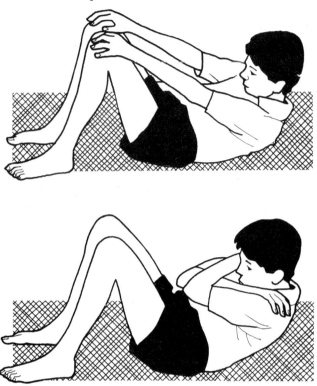

21. **Hip and trunk extensors**: the child lies prone, with hands held behind the head, elbows off the floor, lifts the head and shoulders and one leg upwards, keeping the knee of the moving leg absolutely straight, lowers down, then lifts the head and shoulders and the other leg upwards. You record any difficulty in achieving the movement, or failure to maintain full extension (straightness) in the moving leg's knee. You can then test muscle endurance by counting the repetitions achieved over thirty seconds or one minute.

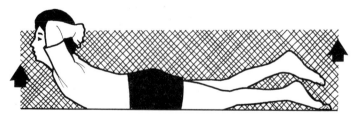

22. **Chest muscle power**: this can be measured by asking the child to hold a 'Bullworker' at arm's length and then to press inwards as hard as possible, so that you can read off the movement achieved on the measuring scale. If you repeat the test three times, you can take the highest reading, but you should note which of the three attempts it is.

23. **Shoulders**: standing up straight, and looking straight forwards, the child lifts the arms up sideways with elbows straight and palms facing downwards, keeping the neck muscles relaxed. You note whether the neck muscles (*trapezii*) contract before the arms reach the horizontal. Then you check whether the child is able to control any tension in the neck muscles by asking him or her to tense then relax the neck muscles while keeping the arms held out sideways.

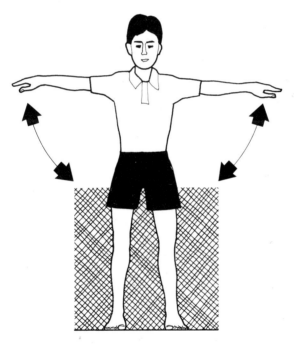

24. **Shoulder elevation stretch**: the child stands with back to a wall, with feet, seat, shoulders and head in contact with the wall, and lifts both arms straight backwards above the head towards the wall. You note whether the child touches the wall easily, keeping the rest

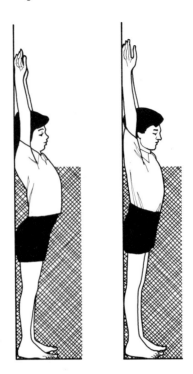

of his or her body in contact, or you measure how far from the wall the middle fingers are. You should also note whether the child arches the back in order to achieve hand contact with the wall.

25. **Shoulders and arms**: the child is asked to clap his/her hands together rapidly, firstly alternating in front of and behind the body; secondly overhead and behind the back. Repetitions are counted over thirty seconds or one minute, and any hesitation or difficulty is noted.

26. **Shoulder rotation flexibility**: the child, standing, puts one hand behind his or her back, with the elbow fully bent to bring the arm up towards the shoulder blades. The other arm is stretched upwards, with the elbow bent to bring the arm behind the head and down towards the shoulder blades. The child then tries to touch the hands together. You note how much the fingers overlap if they meet, or how far apart the middle fingers are, if not.

27. **Forearm stretch**: the child holds one arm straight forwards, palm up, and draws the fingers back with the other hand, keeping the

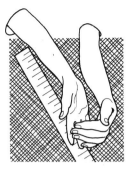

elbow straight. You measure the distance between the middle finger tip and the bony tip at the back of the elbow (*olecranon process*), then repeat the test on the other arm.

28. **Finger dexterity**: the child is asked to touch the thumb to each finger of its own hand in turn, in quick succession, over thirty seconds or one minute, each complete sequence counting as one repetition. The repetitions are counted for each hand, and any noticeable difficulty of co-ordination noted.

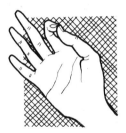

29. **Little finger control**: the child is asked to move the little finger sideways to touch a marker, keeping the other fingers

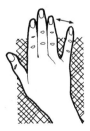

completely still, and the hand straight in line with the arm. The hand is placed palm down on a table, then the test is repeated with the palm facing upwards. Count the repetitions achieved over fifteen or thirty seconds on each hand in turn in each position. Only accurate movements count.

30. **Grip strength**: this can be measured using one of the standard dynamometers.

Checklist for injury prevention

- Choose the child's sports carefully: give the child opportunities for varied exercise activities, if possible.
- Try to choose small-scale versions of sports for young children, such as mini-rugby or short tennis.
- Monitor the child, watching to see if he or she is struggling while doing a particular activity.
- Stop the child from doing too much of one sport, especially if he or she is spending too much time on it every day, or looking tired and drawn.
- When a child starts a new sport, let him or her learn it in easy, progressive stages spread out over days or weeks.
- Give the child the chance to learn sports techniques properly, through a good teacher or coach, if you cannot teach basic skills yourself.
- Allow for the child's growth phases, and be prepared to reduce the child's sport during active growth periods.
- Keep a record of the child's height, weight and shoe size, until the child is old enough to do this independently.
- If in doubt about whether a child should be doing a particular sport, ask the advice of a professional coach, chartered physiotherapist or sports doctor.
- Always make sure that children are adequately supervised during sports.
- Teach the child the rules and safety practices involved in a game.
- Always check that the environment is safe before allowing children to start playing games.
- Make sure that the child is properly dressed for the sport and the conditions, with the right type of shoes, and that all clothing fits well.
- Make sure the child's sports equipment is the correct size for the child's stage of development.

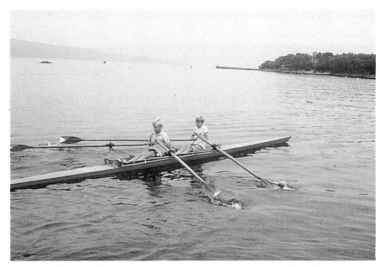

Water skills for rowing are best learned young, in a sculling boat.

• Make sure the child has efficient protective equipment, where the sport requires it.

• Make sure any physical fitness training is appropriate for the child's stage of development.

• If the training is background work for a sport, make sure the programme is properly tailored to the sport, and that it allows for rest and recovery.

• If possible, have the child monitored physiologically and biomechanically at regular intervals, especially if he or she is involved in competitive sport.

• Encourage the child to do any recommended remedial exercises properly and regularly.

• Never allow any child to play games or sports when in pain or unwell.

• If you are not sure whether the child is fit enough to resume sport after an injury or illness, have him or her checked by a chartered physiotherapist or your doctor.

• If you are worried about the child's medical fitness, ask your doctor or the school medical officer to assess the child and judge whether he or she should be doing sport or a particular game.

• Set out realistic goals for the child, using encouragement, not direct pressure, whether the child is involved in competitive sport or exercise for health.

7 Bone Injuries

Children's bones form the basic support structure allowing mechanical movements.[1] Before birth, the bones are mainly formed in soft cartilage, and they gradually transform into hard bones. The process is called *ossification*, and bone growth happens from *centres of ossification*.[2] The long bones which form the arms and legs consist of a central shaft called the *diaphysis*, expanded ends called *epiphyses*, and the physis, a layer of cartilage between the two which is also called the *epiphyseal plate*, *growth plate* or *growth cartilage*. The *metaphysis* is the end part of the diaphysis, where the long bone shaft meets the growth cartilage. Where a tendon joins onto a bone there is usually a special attachment 'knob' called an *apophysis*, which forms separately from the rest of the bone. The separate parts of each bone gradually grow together and harden into the final mature shape in a process called *fusion*. As the bones grow, the child develops height and breadth, accompanied by a change in body proportions. Bone development is extremely complicated, because centres of ossification appear at different times in different bones, but they do not develop at a uniform rate, nor in order of appearance. They fuse at different ages, and the process is generally slightly quicker in girls than boys. The whole bone growth process is not complete until the child reaches the age of about 20–25.

Injuries involving the bones are probably the most important category of children's sports injuries. Although the causes of children's bone injuries can be similar to those of adults, growing bone may react to the damage in a different way from mature bone. Not only is there damage at the time to the body's support structure, but these injuries can also affect the subsequent growth of the bone(s) involved. Traumatic injuries can cause excessive loading on

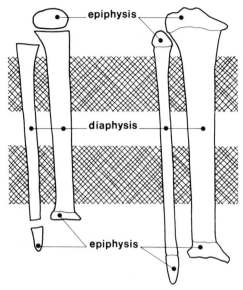

Bone growth: long bones like the fibula and tibia form in separate parts (left) which then fuse together into their mature shapes.

a bone, so that the bone cracks or breaks. The bone(s) involved can be damaged by bending, twisting or crushing forces. Overuse injuries can cause an attritional overload against a bone. The stresses on bones are technically termed compression and tension loads, and bone fractures have been defined as the bone's failure to store enough energy through temporary deformation (such as giving or bending), to withstand the load offered against the bone: therefore the bone gives way.[3]

The definitions of the basic types of bone fracture are similar to adult classifications. A *closed* fracture is a bone break without damage to the overlying skin. An *open* or *compound* fracture involves a skin wound. A *simple* fracture has only one break, whereas a *comminuted* fracture is a shattered bone. A *complicated* fracture means that other structures, like nerves or blood vessels, have been damaged together with the bone. An *avulsion* fracture happens when a tendon is put under major stress and, instead of tearing itself, shears off the knob of bone to which it is attached. A *stress* fracture is a crack or break in a bone caused by gradual overload through repetitive pressure against the bone. The types of fractures which only happen to children are *greenstick* fractures, in which the bone cracks and bends instead of breaking right through, because of its pliability; and *metaphyseal*, *physeal* and *epiphyseal* fractures, which involve the growth areas of the bones.

Traumatic fractures

Any traumatic bone fracture in a child, whether obvious or only suspected, must be treated properly and professionally, preferably by an orthopaedic consultant specializing in paediatrics (children's treatment).[4] If a child suffers a bad knock or fall, and does not get back into action spontaneously, responsible adults should treat the injury as a possible bone fracture, and have the child transferred to the hospital as quickly as possible. Sometimes the signs of bone damage, such as swelling, bruising and localized pain, are only slight, and take some moments to show up, so one should not be in too much of a hurry to get the child up or back into the game. If the injury happens close to a joint such as the ankle, knee or elbow, it may be tempting to assume that the damage is a simple 'joint sprain'. However, you should remember that the joints are formed where the bone ends meet, and the bone ends are the sites of bone growth. Depending on the age of the child, the growth area of the bone may be more vulnerable to shearing stresses than the joint's ligaments and muscles, so in many cases you are more likely to be dealing with a potentially serious growth plate (epiphyseal) fracture than a soft tissue tear alone.[5, 6]

In the hip region, a major complication called *slipped capital femoral epiphysis* can happen following trauma to the upper end of the thigh-bone (femur). The rounded head of the bone slips backwards and downwards on the femoral neck, either suddenly or gradually. This causes a deformity which affects the hip joint movement, and gives pain which may be felt in the groin region, although the pain is often referred to the knee without any evident soreness in the hip itself. Sometimes, especially in the very young child, there is little apparent pain, but the child limps without knowing why. There may be a painful or painless 'click' when the joint is moved in certain ways. The slipped capital epiphysis has been recorded as happening at any stage between the ages of 8 and 17, with boys more vulnerable than girls.[7] The cause of the slippage is disruption in the bone's growth plate, and this is usually present before the accident which finds the weakness. For this reason, the slippage can happen even after only slight damage to the thigh-bone. The exact cause of the growth plate damage often remains unknown, although it can be the result of repeated minor injuries. The surgeon usually operates to correct the bone distortion, and the child is then monitored carefully towards full recovery. As this injury carries a strong risk of leading to early degenerative arthritis (osteoarthritis), sometimes before the age of 30, early and accurate diagnosis and treatment are essential.

When a fracture happens close to a joint, apart from the threat to the epiphysis, there is a risk that the bone's cartilage covering within the joint can be damaged. This is called an *osteochondral fracture*. Bone cartilage (as distinct from the soft-tissue cartilages found, for instance, in the knee) forms a smooth, hard-wearing surface over the bone ends inside moving (synovial) joints.[1] When it is damaged, particles can be broken off. If they shear off completely, they become loose bodies in the joint. The damage may not be obvious at first, but can show up weeks or months later, when the child complains of localized pain in the joint, accompanied by swelling, and sometimes a feelings of locking or giving way when the joint is in a certain position.

Osteochondritis dissecans is a particular type of damage to bone cartilage which happens most commonly at the lower end of the thigh-bone within the knee joint,[8, 9] but can happen in other joints, such as the ankle.[10] A fragment of the bone cartilage, sometimes with part of the bone underneath, becomes detached from the underlying bone. At the knee, this causes a defect in the knuckle of the thigh-bone, although the fragment may or may not shear off completely. The condition can happen without causing any noticeable symptoms, but otherwise the result is stiffness, swelling, soreness, clicking, locking and/or giving way at the knee. It can be the result of trauma, but it is also thought to happen for a variety of other reasons. It is most common in teenagers aged between 14 and 16, but has been known in children as young as 4. Minor osteochondral damage can heal naturally, so the child may only need a period of reduced sports, while the joint may be protected in a splint or plaster cast for six to eight weeks to allow healing to take place. However, if there are loose bodies floating in the joint as a result of the damage, surgery is usually needed to remove the fragments or re-attach them in place. In all cases, the child should have a period of remedial exercises before resuming normal sports.

Special care is needed if the child's head has been hit, even if there is no sign of concussion.[11] On no account should the child be allowed to continue playing. It is wise to take the child to hospital. At the very least, the child should be kept at rest for a day or two, and watched in case any signs of brain damage or head injury show up in the hours following the accident. A skull fracture may not be obvious at first: the danger is that any accompanying bleeding can press on the brain and damage it. Tell-tale warning signs of internal damage following a blow to the head are bleeding or light-coloured fluid coming from the ears or nose, or heavy bruising appearing round the eyes.

If a traumatic injury involves a probable fracture in the back or neck, the child should not be moved until professional help is at hand, in case there is damage to the spinal cord which could cause paralysis in the arms and legs. Less severe injuries can cause 'trapped nerves', giving feeling of referred pain or odd sensations in the legs if the damage is in the lower back, or in the arms if the neck has been hurt. The child must be guided through recovery with professional medical help. After any notable spinal injury to a child, responsible adults have to consider carefully whether the child should be allowed to return at all to high-risk sports such as rugby, gymnastics, motorbike scrambling and high jumping.

If any broken bone is accompanied by a skin wound, the cut should be covered with a sterile dressing, and the child taken to hospital as an emergency. When a child has a compound fracture, there is a particular risk that *osteomyelitis* (inflammation of the bone marrow) can develop. This is a serious condition which can be fatal, although correctly applied antibiotics can control it.

The surgeon's treatment of any traumatic fracture aims to provide the correct alignment of the bone, as in adult fracture treatment, but the surgeon also has to take into account any bone growth problems which might arise as a result of the damage. This is especially important if the fracture affects the growing end of a bone. Technically, metaphyseal, physeal and epiphyseal fractures have been classified according to the distinct patterns in which they tend to occur.[12] Damage to the growth plate can stunt the bone's growth. On the other hand, shaft fractures in a long bone like the thigh-bone (femur) can make the bone grow too long. It may be necessary for the surgeon to monitor the child's progress for several years after a major fracture. While a bad fracture with complications may need surgery and sometimes prolonged in-patient hospital treatment, a simple fracture in a very young (pre-teen) child may only need

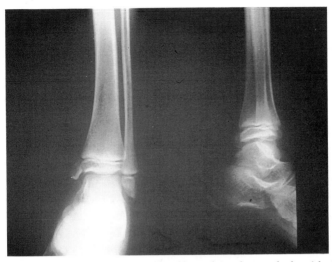

*Fracture of the medial malleolus at the ankle involving the growth plate (physis),
which is at special risk of early closure.*
(Photograph courtesy of the London Hospital).

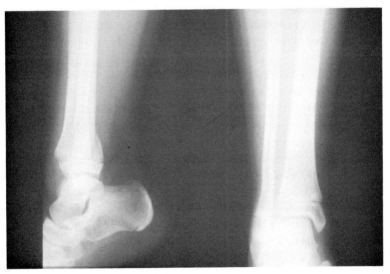

A Type II fracture at the back of the tibia, close to the ankle joint.
(Photograph courtesy of the London Hospital).

support for a relatively short time, while the bone heals and remodels itself. The surgeon's treatment depends on the type of the traumatic fracture; the age of the child; and the presence or absence of potentially dangerous complications.

Once a fracture has healed, the child should receive rehabilitation treatment. Paediatric surgeons or physicians often assume that the child will recover normal function spontaneously, especially if the child is very young and the fracture has healed quickly and without complications. It is true that children manage to compensate very well for a body part which is temporarily out of action. For instance, a child usually has no problems coping with crutches and hopping around with a leg in plaster. However, the weakness which occurs because the limb has been out of action for a period usually lasts for several weeks after apparent recovery, so the compensating muscles continue to overwork, even though the imbalance may not be obvious enough to cause a visible disability or limp. If the muscles are not re-strengthened and stretched through accurate remedial exercises, perhaps combined with electrical muscle stimulation, there is a risk that even a slight residual imbalance will contribute to secondary problems sooner or later. For instance, lack of rehabilitation for a leg fracture may make the child more vulnerable to knee or hip problems, either in the injured leg, or as the result of overload in the compensating leg; a hand fracture might cause later problems in the elbow or shoulder. These effects may be delayed for several years: a fracture sustained at the age of 6 might contribute to subsequent injury in the mid-teen period.

Stress fractures

Stress fractures are overuse injuries which happen in the same way in children as they do in adults.[13] They can happen at any age, and have been reported in children as young as 3,[14] although they are said to be unusual in children under the age of 10.[15] A stress fracture is a bone crack caused by continual repetitive pressure from a muscle, muscle group or tendon pulling against a bone. Any bone in the body which is subject to pressure from a muscle or tendon can be cracked through this type of subtle excessive loading. The bone is essentially healthy, although there may be background factors making it more prone to stress injury. For instance, the child may have a congenital 'defect', such as a bipartite or tripartite patella, in which the parts of the knee-cap have failed to fuse together properly,

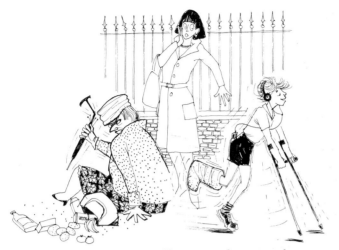

Children may have no problems getting about on crutches.

or a spondylolysis, in which the strut of a spinal bone is similarly separated from its main bone. It is possible that dietary deficiencies can play a part in weakening the child's bones generally and making them more vulnerable to injuries due to repetitive pressure. It is also suspected that girls with menstrual problems such as amenorrhoea (lack of periods) may be more susceptible to stress fractures.

The stress fracture is very different from a traumatic fracture, in that there is no episode of accident or injury, and the first signs of bone damage are very subtle. There may be slight redness of the skin, and possibly some swelling. The child might complain of localized pain or just an ache. The pain may be felt only at night, after sport, or it may be noticeable during sport. The muscles over the bone might go into spasm, giving a feeling of muscle pull, tightness or cramp. There may be an obvious limp, or, if the arm is affected, the child may avoid using it. The pain always eases with a few days' rest from sport, but it returns quickly once the causative sport is resumed.

As the stress fracture is specifically the result of repetitive movement, it is an in-built risk in sports like rowing and long-distance running. Stress fractures in the spinal bones are relatively common among weightlifters, divers, rowers, hockey players and gymnasts.[16, 17] If the crack occurs in one of the struts (*pars interarticularis*) which lies behind the body of a vertebra and forms its connexion with the next vertebra, it is called a spondylolysis.[18] This is a condition which can also be present congenitally (from birth) without necessarily causing pain, except when irritated by certain activities. Whether congenital or acquired, once the bone is painful, it is treated in the same way as any other stress fracture: painful activities are avoided, painless exercises or sports encouraged. Sometimes a special brace is used to protect the spine.[19] If the struts on both sides of a vertebra are cracked by repetitive stress, the body of the bone usually slips forward relative to the other vertebrae: this is called a spondylolisthesis.[20] Surgery may be needed to stabilize the bones. Spondylolysis and spondylolisthesis are specially common in older teenagers, and they usually happen in the lower half of the spine.

In runners, stress fractures tend to happen in the foot- and leg-bones, especially the lower part of the shin-bone (tibia) and outer leg-bone (fibula), although they can happen in the thigh-bone and as far up as the pelvic bones. Sports which are varied by nature can still carry similar risks of stress fractures if certain patterns of movement predominate, or if certain movements are practised on a repetitive basis. For instance, sports involving constant knee-bending, such as squash and skiing, put the knee-cap at special risk of stress fractures. Gymnasts can damage the wrist, elbow or arm-bones through overdoing a single pattern of movement involving hand-stands or vaults; tennis players can damage bones in the arm, ribs or spine through intensive practice of a single stroke like the serve; and players of all sports can put themselves at risk of stress fractures through repetitive-movement fitness training like skipping and running.

Diagnosis is a matter for the specialist. The doctor may have to exclude more serious types of bone condition, such as a tumour, infection or osteomyelitis. Stress fractures are difficult to identify on X-ray, except when the bone is healing, or if it has broken completely, so other tests such as bone scans may be done, if necessary. The story of how the pain started is invaluable in helping to establish whether or not the problem might be a stress fracture. Typically, there is a history of an increase in a repetitive activity: the child may have been taken on a long hike over several days, or started intensive running training, or practised drills during a squad training weekend, or increased sports practice in preparation for a competition. Sometimes the problem arises when the child resumes sport too enthusiastically after a break for illness or a holiday. The description of the child's activities and pain pattern are usually sufficient to indicate whether the problem is a stress fracture. The responsible adult can help to tell the story, but it is also important to allow the child to describe what has happened, partly to give the child a sense of involvement, and partly because children often remember important details which may have been missed by the adults.

Once the stress fracture has been diagnosed, it needs time in order to heal. Occasionally, surgery is needed, if there are displaced bone fragments, or if the bone does not heal despite proper care. Otherwise, the damaged bone is usually not put into a plaster cast, because total immobilization tends to weaken the bone further and to prevent healing. For a spondylolisthesis, a special brace may be used to correct the child's spinal mechanics and prevent further slippage of the vertebra.[21] Sometimes a cast is used to stop the child from causing further damage by continuing normal sports, but then remedial exercises to improve localized muscle tone and stimulate the circulation are essential. If a leg stress fracture causes pain while walking, the child uses crutches until full weight-bearing is comfortable.

Ice is used to relieve any continuing pain and swelling. The chartered physiotherapist may use electrical stimulation to improve the muscle tone around the affected bone without stressing it. Any pain-causing activity has to be avoided, but painless activities, on the contrary, are encouraged. The child may be able to play games using varied movements, and swimming and cycling are usually possible. The 'rest' period has to last for at least four weeks, in the case of a light bone like the fibula or a metatarsal (foot-bone), up to twelve weeks or more for a major weight-bearing bone like the tibia (shin-bone) or femur (thigh-bone). The physiotherapist should set out the exercise programme and monitor the child's progess to full recovery. If necessary, the X-rays or bone scans are repeated at the end of the rest period, to check whether full healing has taken place.

If the pain of a stress fracture is ignored, the damage to the bone gets worse, and in some cases the bone shatters. If this happens, the child needs hospital treatment, and the surgeon may have to operate to fix the broken pieces together, or to remove any fragments which cannot be mended. After the bone has healed, the child is allowed to get back to normal activities in very easy stages.

Stress fractures are preventable, and once one has occurred, it is important to avoid the risk of subsequent secondary stress fractures. The cause of the stress fracture must be identified, and the same mistake avoided in future. Single patterns of muscle pull against certain bones should be avoided, and bone strength should be maximized through a progressive muscle strengthening programme. The following guidelines can help to achieve these aims:

1. The child should recover fully from any injury or illness, before being allowed to resume sport.
2. The child's diet should be analysed, and improved, if necessary. It may be helpful to consult a dietician for detailed advice.
3. For the female with menstrual irregularities, a full medical check-up may need to be followed by biochemical screening from a medical nutritionist, so that any deficiencies in minerals or other necessary substances can be identified and corrected.
4. The child should not be allowed to return to intensive sport too soon after any injury or lay-off. The practitioner's advice on when to re-start should be followed.
5. At least two or three rest days should be allowed between active sports sessions, especially if they involve repetitive movements.
6. The child should always build up sporting activities very gradually, allowing recovery days after any increased training load.
7. Any changes in a sports programme or training schedule should be introduced gradually, again allowing time for recovery.
8. Over-training, particularly through doing sessions on consecutive days, should not be allowed, especially in repetitive sports like running.
9. Other sports or body conditioning training should be used to counteract the stresses of repetitive sports, and to improve overall muscle and bone strength.
10. Even a slight pain felt over a bone during or after sport should never be ignored: the child should not be allowed to return to sport until the pain has been cured. Adults should watch for warning signs, such as a limp or facial expressions of pain.

Apophysitis

Apophysitis is damage to a growth point (apophysis) where a tendon is attached to a bone. There are apophyses close to every major joint, for instance at the back of the heel where the Achilles (calcaneal) tendon is anchored, or just below the knee where the patellar tendon joins the tibial tubercle. Near the hip, some of the gluteal muscles are attached to a knob of bone called the greater trochanter, while the flexor muscle, psoas major, is anchored to the lesser trochanter. At the shoulder, the lesser and greater tuberosities provide the attachment points for several important muscles, while the tendons for the main forearm muscles are attached on either side of the lower end of the arm-bone (humerus). Many apophyses are non-weight-bearing parts within the bigger epiphyses, or growing bone ends. In practice, the terms *epiphysitis* and *apophysitis* are sometimes used interchangeably by doctors to describe this 'growing problem'.[22]

Apophysitis is similar in nature to a stress fracture.[13, 23] It is caused by repetitive strain due to the pressure exerted by a tendon, and it can happen in any apophysis anywhere in the body, just as the stress fracture can occur in any bone subjected to excessive repetitive loading through its attached muscles.[24] Apophysitis is usually an overuse syndrome, and the apophyses tend to be specially vulnerable as they approach and go through their final fusion process of 'glueing' themselves onto their main bones and hardening into their final size and shape. Therefore the teen years are the most vulnerable, with apophysitis tending to happen in specific age groups

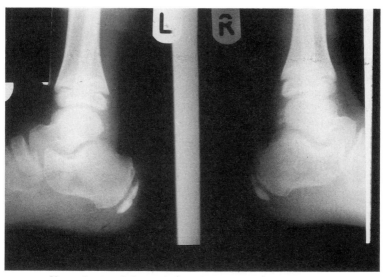

*X-ray showing slight apophysitis of the left heel ('Sever's disease')
in an 11-year-old boy.*

in different areas of the body. In the heel, for instance, calcaneal apophysitis has a special name, *Sever's 'disease'*, and the problem tends to happen between the ages of 10 and 13. At the tibial tubercle just below the knee, the apophysitis is known as *Osgood-Schlatter's 'disease'*, and it usually happens between the ages of 12 and 16.[25] At the lower point (pole) of the knee-cap (patella), repetitive stress through the patellar tendon, especially in the mid-teen years, can cause tiny bone fragments called ossicles to form, and this is called *Sinding-Larsen-Johansson 'disease'*. The iliac crest, over the top of the flank bone just below the waist, is especially vulnerable to apophysitis between the ages of 14 and 17.[26]

The cause of any apophysitis is repetitive stress, repeated minor trauma, or, in a few cases, an episode of more severe traumatic jarring or tension against the bone. As the damage happens when the bone end is specially vulnerable, it is not necessarily due to any increase in sporting activities, and can happen through a normal level of sport (unlike a stress fracture). The site of an apophysitis relates

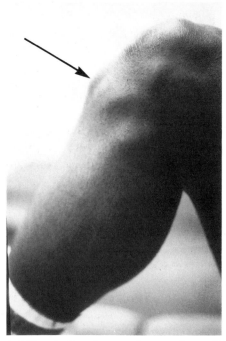

'Osgood-Schlatter's disease' causes a bump at the top of the shin.

directly to the child's sporting activities. Young runners, jumpers, netball and basketball players are specially vulnerable to Sever's 'disease'; runners, footballers, weightlifters and squash players are prone to Osgood-Schlatter's 'disease'. The apophyses at the upper end of the thigh-bone are vulnerable in sports involving kicking, such as karate, American football and rugby. The iliac crest is threatened by sports involving twisting, such as throwing events, hurdling and racket sports. Any of the apophyses of the shoulder or arm can be damaged through gymnastics, racket sports, weightlifting or throwing.

The pain of an apophysitis may be only slight at first, but it gradually gets worse. The child may limp, or guard the injured arm. However, the pain often remains at a fairly low level, so that the child is tempted to continue normal sports. If the child complains at all of pain in one of the 'growth areas', or if adults notice tell-tale signs of injury, the child should be taken to a sports injury specialist. The doctor may diagnose the problem on the basis of the history of excessive or increased sporting activity, and localized tenderness when he presses his fingers over the damaged part of the bone. Otherwise, he may order X-rays to find out whether the growth area has been visibly separated from its main bone.

Treatment for an apophysitis is usually simply rest from any painful, aggravating activities, combined with any form of exercise which can be done without pain. The doctor may immobilize the bone in a plaster cast to stop the child from continuing sport, but this is rarely necessary, if the child, teachers and parents co-operate in restricting the child's sports. Supports may be used, such as bandaging for the knee, wrist or elbow, or shock-absorbing heel cushions. Ice applications can be used for pain relief. A chartered physiotherapist might use electrotherapy for pain relief, but with caution. Some modalities, like ultrasound, are thought to be possibly damaging to the growing epiphysis, and so are considered unsuitable for the treatment of children's bone problems, until further research has proved whether or not this is so.[27] However, the physiotherapist may use electrical stimulation to maintain the muscle function around the injured bone, and the child is always taught appropriate stretching and stabilizing exercises. If the muscles have become very weak, especially round the knee where the muscles are very quickly inhibited by pain, the physiotherapist may teach the child and parents how to use a simple muscle stimulator at home (see p. 161).

The rest phase lasts until the bone is completely pain-free. This may take only a few days, but is more likely to be weeks. If the problem has been allowed to develop to the stage of severe and continuing pain, the problem can take up to two years to resolve, and may leave a permanent visible lump. The lump itself is usually painless once the growth phase has passed, but very occasionally it remains painful when the part is stressed by similar activities to those which caused the problem in the first place. In a very few cases, the child may need surgery to stabilize the bone end, if it has been badly pulled away.

One complication which can happen if the child is allowed to continue normal sports despite the presence of damage at a bone growth point is an *apophyseal avulsion fracture*. The tendon attached to the growth point pulls the bone away completely. This can happen due to repeated stress, but is more likely to occur if a sudden jarring or stretching force is applied to a weakened area, for instance in a blocked tackle or awkward fall. The most common places in which this injury happens are around the pelvis, at the upper end of the thigh-bone (femur), at the lower point (pole) of the knee-cap, and at the tibial tubercle.[28] The pain can be severe if the injury is a sudden traumatic incident, but it can seem deceptively slight if the avulsion is the culmination of cumulative stress.

Surgery may be needed if the specialist feels that the displaced part of the bone is too far out of its proper line. Otherwise, the child is rested, in bed if necessary, until the pain has subsided. After the initial phase, treatment follows the pattern for simple apophysitis and consists of strengthening and stretching exercises, leading to a very gradual return to sport.

Bone conditions and diseases

Diseases can affect bones, like other body tissues, and can cause defects which are not due to accidents or injuries. Sometimes the defect does not cause pain until the child suffers a sports injury in the affected area, so it is only discovered by coincidence. Some children's bone conditions result in visible, painful deformities and growth disturbances. Many of these have been recognized by doctors and surgeons for a long time, and named after the people who first described them, but often their cause is still not understood. In the forefoot, osteochondritis of the second metatarsal head can cause excessive growth, and is called *Freiburg's disease*. In the mid-foot, growth disturbance to the navicular bone is called *Kohler's disease*. At the hip, the femoral head which should form the ball of the joint can fail to grow properly, and this is called *Legg-Calvé-Perthes disease* (often shortened to *Perthes disease*). In the middle (thoracic) part of the spine, the front parts of the vertebral bones can fail to grow, causing wedging of the vertebrae and a pronounced hunched back: this is called *idiopathic kyphosis* or it may be termed *Scheuermann's disease*. Teenagers sometimes develop a pronounced curvature and twist in the spine for no apparent reason, and the name given to this is *idiopathic scoliosis*.

Sport is usually not a causative factor in these conditions, although it can aggravate the pain, if there is any. In each case, the child has to be properly screened and treated by a paediatric specialist, and the responsible adult should ask for as much information as possible about the condition, its treatment, and its possible long-term consequences. The adult should also seek detailed guidance about the most appropriate form of exercise for the child, if any, and the best future pattern of sports. Although most of these conditions have no easy cure, as such, this author considers that remedial exercises are still likely to be appropriate, partly to maintain or improve the blood circulation, and partly to counteract the onset of deformities. In the case of idiopathic scoliosis, for instance, areas of muscle weakness and tightness affecting the length of the spine can be identified and helped by appropriate gentle strengthening and stretching exercises. At the very least, these exercises might improve the child's posture and self-confidence.

8 Soft-Tissue Injuries

While the body's bones are its 'hard tissues', the 'soft tissues', in the sports injuries context, are considered to be those structures which are neither bones nor organs (for instance the heart or the brain). The soft tissues include ligaments, which are specially strengthened bands on a moving joint's enclosing capsule; synovial membranes, which are fluid-forming coverings over moving joints; bursae, or small sacs of synovial fluid designed to allow friction-free movement between two tendons or between a tendon and an underlying bone; fat pads which act as cushions over bones; discs which act as shock absorbers between bones; soft cartilages for shock absorption and free gliding movements in a joint (the knee's menisci are the main examples of these); muscles, which effect the body's movements; and tendons, which are cords connecting the broader muscle bellies to their anchor points on bones, and which are less elastic than muscle.

The growth and development of the soft tissues are dominated by the stages of bone growth. Children vary in structure because of hereditary factors, and there are general differences between races. However, the overall pattern of growth tends to be as follows: up to the age of about 10, the child's muscles are relatively weak but flexible, while the joints, whose bone ends are not fully formed, are reasonably stable but relatively very mobile. In the early teens, the long bones go through the growth spurt, stretching out the muscles that cover them. The muscle-tendon units are lengthened, so they go through a phase of relative weakness and tightness, until they 'catch up' with the bone growth by gaining in bulk and strength. Puberty affects the teenager's development, bringing relative strength gains to boys, coupled with a reduction in body fat, while girls gain fat, especially round the hips, thighs and abdomen (p. 37).

The bone fusion processes that happen mainly in the teenage years tend to reduce the body's flexibility and mobility, as the joints where the bone ends meet become fixed into their final shapes.

At different stages of growth, the child's body alters its proportions. The growing foot is relatively large, compared to the rest of the leg, and it reaches about half of its final length when the child is about 18 months old, while the rest of the leg grows more slowly, reaching half its final length by about 4 years and full length by about the age of 14 in girls, 16 in boys.[1] While boys become broader in the chest and shoulders following puberty, girls broaden at the hips, so the male and female body contours show their divergence at this period of development. As the adolescent approaches full growth, his or her final body shape will depend on the basic build (the balance between tissues like muscles and fat), which is inherited, but is also influenced by diet and exercise habits.

All the soft tissues can be injured through trauma or overuse, just as in the adult. Young children seem to recover quickly from trauma such as knocks and bruises. Traumatic injuries to children of all ages carry the risk that they involve the bone growth plates, so no significant twisting or jarring injury to a joint should be diagnosed as simply a 'sprain' without a doctor checking the bones for damage.[2] Overuse injuries are recognized as an increasing problem among young sports participants, and they are particularly likely among adolescents who specialize in a particular sport and follow intensive training regimes.[3] Teenagers may seem to take longer than expected to recover from supposedly simple muscle strains. This may happen because the teenager is trying to ignore the problem, rather than getting the correct treatment and advice, or because the injury has damaged a bone as well as the muscle, or because the teenager's diet is inadequate, especially if it is deficient in essential minerals or vitamins.

As with bone injuries, the most important aspect of children's soft-tissue injuries is the effect they have on the body's function. Although less serious than bone injuries, soft-tissue injuries always cause *inhibition*, or inability to make full use of the affected area. If this is not corrected through accurate exercise therapy, the child is left with a deficit of movement, strength and/or mobility, which may cause continuing stresses in related parts of the body. These stresses, in turn, can cause secondary injuries, either soon after the original injury, or years later. Treatment for any injury aims to allow the child to exercise correctly, as a prelude to returning to sport. This is an important principle in the treatment of adults' injuries, and should not be neglected when dealing with children's injuries, just because they *appear* to mend easily. The treatment methods themselves are usually kept as simple as possible, avoiding any techniques which carry any risk at all of disrupting bone growth (p. 129). Biomechanical monitoring, to make sure that full functional recovery has been achieved after any injury, is essential. The basic tests described for the child's physical assessment are useful for this purpose, although there are, of course, many more possible tests relating to the detailed specific injuries the child might incur.

The foot and leg

The foot is the child's base of support, and its healthy development is essential for comfort and efficiency when walking, running, jumping or kicking a ball. The contours of the feet vary, mainly through hereditary factors. Feet are very much influenced by shoes: tight and badly fitting shoes can hinder bone growth and create deformities in the toes, besides causing black toe-nails and skin calluses or blisters. Toe-nails can cause pain and therefore alter the foot mechanics, if they are cut badly, or allowed to grow too long so that they catch in the shoes. Rigid shoes can over-stretch the ligaments in the sole of the foot: new shoes tend to be relatively stiff, so they should always be 'broken in' before the child wears them for any length of time, or for serious exercise. The small muscles which control the feet are developed by exercise, especially if it is done barefoot, and involves active movements for the toes.

The child may have 'flat feet', in which the main arch is low to the ground, so that most of the sole of the foot touches the ground. If the child has high arches, the feet are curved upwards, pulled by tight tendons over the top (*dorsum*) and under the mid-foot, resulting in the central area and inner side of the sole being held off the ground. The child may have a hereditary tendency to bunions, in which the big toe is pulled over by shortened, tight tendons towards the other toes on the same foot, creating a visible lump at the side of the ball of the foot.

The orientation of the feet has an effect on the ankle, knee and pelvic joints.[4] If the foot flattens excessively during walking or running, stress is created along the inner side of the heel, ankle, Achilles tendon, lower leg and knee. Technically, this is called *over-pronation*, and it can contribute to strains in the muscles, tendons and ligaments where they are over-stretched. If the foot turns outwards too much, in *over-supination*, there are extra stresses on the outer side of the leg and knee. The high-arched foot may be a poor shock absorber, so that the normal jarring of running, jumping or kicking creates excessive stress on the foot, ankle, leg or knee. Bunions can distort the normal load-bearing area of the feet away from the ball of the foot towards the outer part of the forefoot. In normal situations, foot variations may not cause any problems. However, they can become important factors in injuries if the child is doing a lot of sport, or if the shoes worn are inappropriate to the child's feet.

Foot development depends on the balance between the efficiency of the small muscles in the feet themselves (the *intrinsics*) and that of the longer muscles and their tendons which link the lower leg to the foot and toe bones. Flat feet, for instance, can be due to weakness in the intrinsic muscles, or to inefficiency in the long lower leg muscles. Intrinsic muscle weakness is usually due to lack of sufficient exercise, for instance if the child sits around most of the time, or wears tight shoes for walking and sports. Relative weakness in the lower leg muscles can be hereditary. Some children, for example, take after one parent in making their first steps relatively late, even though they can crawl and move about without difficulty. The child may be able to pull him or herself up into standing by using the arms, but will be unable to balance and move one leg at a time, preferring to move around on all fours for speed. This late start in walking may be carried through, so that the child is slow at running, appearing flat-footed, and perhaps even suffering pain when he or she runs or jumps. The foot may be very mobile, with a good arch when the child stands still, but it flattens during weight-bearing movements when the child stands and balances or tries to go up and down on the toes, because the lower leg muscles are weak.

Painful feet can put children off sport, especially if they are forced to continue games and gymnastics when they are very young, despite their complaints. Sometimes the child notices pain in both feet on running or jumping, especially barefoot. The pains may be related to injury, especially to the long plantar ligament or the plantar fascia, two strong binding tissues under the sole, or to the bones of the foot. However, it is relatively unusual for injury to happen to both feet at the same time. Occasionally, the foot pain is a symptom of an arthritic condition (which may be inherited within the family). Often, however, the foot pain has no identifiable cause, beyond weakness in the intrinsic foot muscles or the lower leg muscles. In some children, the feet are painful even at rest, perhaps in bed at night, or when the child is sitting still. These pains may start when the child is very young, possibly 2 or 3, and then persist until the teenage years. The pains may disappear quite suddenly at any stage in the child's growth.

Any foot pain should, of course, be checked by the child's doctor to establish whether it is due to injury or disease, so that appropriate treatment can be given. If the pain is functional, you may have to buy the child new, more appropriate shoes. Cushioned insoles may be needed as well. If the foot mechanics need correcting, a physiotherapist or podiatrist may assess the child's feet, and make up specially fitted arch or heel supports (orthotics) to try to correct the foot's directions of movement. If this is done, they have to be re-checked at frequent intervals, as the child's foot can change its movements during growth, and the foot naturally gets bigger. If any of the muscles are weak, the physiotherapist will teach the child appropriate exercises, and may use electrical stimulation to help the muscles to work more efficiently: the toes should be able to flatten to the floor, and spread out sideways, and the big toe should be able to move independently of the others. The child should also be able to walk on the toes, heels and edges of the feet without pain or difficulty. Balance exercises are important as a measure of the child's co-ordination from the foot upwards, so the child may have to practise balancing on one leg, and standing one-legged on the wobble board (see p. 100, test exercises 1–3).

The ankle can be sprained when it is over-twisted, over-compressed or over-stretched in any direction. The cause can be a fall, or a sliding, awkward or blocked movement. It can relate directly

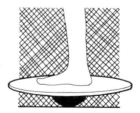

Balancing on the wobble board.

to inappropriate shoes, such as thick-soled trainers worn for court games involving sudden twists and turns. The ankle joint may be injured on its own, but there is often involvement of the joints in the hindfoot under the ankle. Especially in young children, the possibility of damage to the bone growth plates has to be ruled out before the diagnosis of a soft-tissue sprain is made, because the ankle ligaments are stronger than its bones up to the age of about 15.[5] Any ankle injury in a child, teenager or adult spoils the normal co-ordination of the joint, because the joint's nerves are inevitably damaged together with the soft tissues such as the ligaments, capsule or tendon. When a child seems to have so-called 'weak ankles', which are repeatedly being sprained even under only minor stresses, the weakness relates to poor co-ordination and balance mechanisms (technically called *proprioception*), rather than to weak muscles alone. Therefore, the nerves have to be re-trained through co-ordination exercises such as balancing on the wobble board (p. 100, test exercise 1; also test exercises 2–4).

Taping the ankle to give it firm support may be necessary in the early stages of recovery from a sprain, to prevent further injuries such as might happen when the child is walking on uneven pavements, or if he or she turns suddenly and catches the ankle. In the United States, especially, taping the ankles is often done routinely in sports like basketball, gymnastics and American football, and this has been shown to reduce the numbers of sprained ankles among sports players.[6] However, this author considers that binding the whole joint with inelastic bandaging as a prophylactic measure against ankle sprains is inadvisable. I believe that taping which reduces the ankle's mobility is likely to weaken the joint, and throw stress upwards to the knee, pelvis and lower back during jumping and landing, or running and changing direction quickly.

It has been shown that the inelastic taping tends to slacken after a short period, losing some of its supportiveness, and it is also thought that elastic support bandaging might be as effective as non-stretch taping, if not more so.[7] It is increasingly accepted that the most important effect of ankle taping is to stimulate the nerves to the ankle's controlling tendons and ligaments by stretching the skin where it is attached. This reinforces the ankle's own protective mechanisms. Taping should not be a substitute for a remedial exercise programme to improve the joint's co-ordination. For injury prevention, balance exercises and wobble board work should be a routine part of background training for sports such as basketball, netball and gymnastics. Physical education lessons should also include as many exercises involving the balance mechanisms as possible.

During recovery from an ankle injury, the child might limp, and this has to be corrected. The foot movements may be altered, so the physiotherapist may teach the child foot and toe exercises, and may help the muscle work with electrical stimulation. The foot may even need orthotic support, fitted by the physiotherapist or podiatrist, to make it work properly again. If the child's shoes were inappropriate, or badly worn down, especially round the heel or heel counter, new shoes may also be needed.

The calf muscles and their attached Achilles tendon are the main muscles on the back of the lower leg. They can be injured during sports involving rapid movements, such as squash, badminton and football. Traumatic tears or part-tears are very rare in young children, but more likely to happen in older teenagers. In children of all ages, friction from badly designed shoes is a major cause of irritation to the lower end of the Achilles tendon, just above the back of the ankle, and pressure from high backed shoes or boots can contribute to tears in any part of the calf and Achilles structure.[8] Poor cushioning, especially in the heel of the shoe, can also contribute to calf injuries. Fatigue is an important factor in calf muscle and Achilles tendon tears. Insufficient fluid intake can cause calf cramps, which in turn can lead to muscle tears. Muscle weakness can contribute to nagging 'growing pains' in the calf muscles, and this is especially likely to happen to the child who started walking relatively late as a baby.

Calf muscle injuries cause tightness in the back of the lower leg, which also affects the knee by preventing it from straightening out fully. Flexibility has to be regained through passive stretching exercises (p. 101, numbers 5 and 11). Equally importantly, once the injury pain has subsided, the child has to work on remedial exercises to restore full calf efficiency. As well as being able to go up and down on the toes with the knees straight (p. 101, test exercise 4), the child should practise the balance and co-ordination test exercises (p. 100, test exercises 1 and 3). In the later stages of recovery, the combined exercise for calf efficiency is used (p. 102, test exercise 6), and the child should practise going up and down on the ball of the foot with the toes held up off the floor, first on both feet together, then on the recovering leg alone. Before returning to normal sports, full stretch and strength should be regained, and the child should be able to hop, skip, and sprint, in various directions. Following any calf or Achilles tendon injury, all the child's shoes should be carefully checked, and modified or replaced as necessary.

The anterior tibial muscles on the front of the lower leg act to draw the foot upwards at the ankle, while the peroneal muscles on the outer side of the leg pull the foot outwards. The muscles can be injured through over-strain or sudden shearing stresses, causing small or large tears. The compartment syndrome is a relatively common problem in the anterior tibial muscles, although the condition can happen in other muscle groups throughout the body:[9] the muscle swells within its containing sheath (fascia), or excess fluid accumulates, causing constriction and pain during exercise, which is relieved immediately afterwards, especially if ice or cold compresses are applied to the area. If the problem occurs suddenly and severely, it should be treated as an emergency, as the blood flow through the muscles may be cut off (this is technically called *ischaemia*). In most cases, the syndrome is treated by rest from normal sport, especially running, coupled with physiotherapy treatment, which might include slow-pulse electrical stimulation for the affected muscles. If the problem persists, surgery may be needed to release the tight muscle sheath.

Injury to any of the muscles or tendons controlling the foot from the lower leg can upset the balance which holds the foot and ankle in proper alignment. If the child limps to avoid putting pressure through the injured area, the foot may work with over-pronation, and may be loaded awkwardly through being rolled across its width instead of through its length as the child walks. The false leverage created through the leg muscles then creates further problems of muscle imbalance by over-stretching some of the muscles and shortening others. If the child is limping badly because of a muscle or tendon injury, the leg should be supported with comfortable bandaging, and the child should use crutches to keep the pressure off the leg. In the recovering phases, full co-ordination must be regained, so all the co-ordination exercises mentioned for ankle and calf injuries should be practised until they can be performed perfectly.

The thigh

Thigh muscle injuries are relatively uncommon in very young children. They are more likely to occur when the child is approaching the teenage period. The growth spurt makes the thigh-bone (femur) grow longer, and the angle at which the end of the bone lies in contact with the shin-bone (tibia) becomes narrower because the thigh-bone is no longer held turned as far forward as in early childhood. This angle is technically termed *femoral version*: if the thigh-bone is held further forward than normal, it is described as *medial femoral torsion*, while an unusually reduced hip angle relative to the shin-bone is called *lateral femoral torsion*.[10] The angle at which the thigh-bones lie affects the pelvic joints, hips, knees and often the feet as well. If both the thigh- and shin-bones turn inwards, the child is likely to appear pigeon-toed. If the thigh-bone is rotated inwards with a compensating outward twist of the shin-bone at the knee, the child may seem knock-kneed.

After the growth spurt and puberty, the thigh-bone lies more vertically in boys than in girls. Girls develop a broader pelvis to allow for childbearing, so their hips are set wider apart and their thigh-bones are angled inwards towards the knees. As the thigh-bone gains in length, its covering muscles are stretched out, becoming relatively weak and tight. This phase may, unfortunately, coincide with a period when the growing child is increasingly active. The young teenager may be playing a wide variety of sports at school, or perhaps starting to join in specialized sport for competition.

Any injury or pain in the thigh muscles is likely to affect the movements and freedom of the knee or hip, or both. There may also be associated stresses affecting the lower back, abdominal muscles, lower leg, ankle and foot. If the quadriceps muscles on the front of the thigh are injured, the knee-cap joint may become stiff, leading to tightness in the patellar tendon which links the knee-cap to the shin-bone. This can be an indirect cause of injury to the front of the knee, including knee-cap joint pain, subluxation or dislocation, or patellar tendon strain (p. 157). Injury causing spasm and shortening in the long muscles over the front of the thigh (sartorius and rectus femoris) can cause tightness not only over the knee but also over the front of the hip. This might draw the hip forwards and limit its backward and rotary movements, which in turn can increase the forward curve (lordosis) of the lower back on that side. Therefore significant imbalance is caused, which can result in secondary injuries in the hip or lower back either on the injured side or the opposite side, through overloading.

Treatment for the muscles on the front of the thigh is always conservative: any deep or energetic massage in the early stages of recovery carries the risk of causing bone formation in the muscles (*myositis ossificans*),[11] in children as in adults. If the thigh muscles have been injured by a direct blow or kick (often called a 'Charley-horse' injury), there is a risk of myositis ossificans forming anyway, so treatment aims to prevent further abnormal bone development, and to encourage the extra bone to be absorbed. If myositis ossificans does occur, the bone is usually not removed surgically. With or without myositis ossificans, the aim of treatment is to regain full stretch and strength in the front thigh muscles through remedial exercises before the child returns to sport.[12] Quadriceps muscle function can be assessed simply through the test exercises 8 and 9 (p. 103), or more accurately on sophisticated computerized muscle measuring apparatus such as the Kin Com, Lido or Cybex.

The hamstring muscles on the back of the thigh can be strained or torn in traumatic or overuse injuries, such as a sudden tear while sprinting, or gradual pain linked with longer-distance running. As they are attached to the seat bone at their upper end, and behind the knee at the lower end, tightness and weakness in them can affect the calf, hip, pelvic joints and lower back, or the knee's balance of movements. Conversely, problems in these areas can contribute to hamstring injuries. A muscle imbalance in which the quadriceps group is relatively much stronger than the hamstrings on the same leg is an important factor leading to hamstring injuries.[13, 14] If the hamstrings are injured repeatedly, which is a problem young sprinters often have, the calf muscles build up to compensate for the inefficiency in the hamstrings, and this can lead to lower leg or knee problems.

Full flexibility of the hamstring muscles is maintained or regained through passive stretching exercises. However, over-stretching is a common cause of hamstring muscle strain in teenagers. Following the growth spurt, the child may no longer be able to touch his or her toes while standing up; encouraging the child to keep trying to do this can strain or tear the hamstrings. In the older teenager and adult, forced toe-touching can cause back strain, sometimes complicated by a hamstring strain or nerve pain referred to the hamstring region from the back. Therefore, passive stretching for the ham-

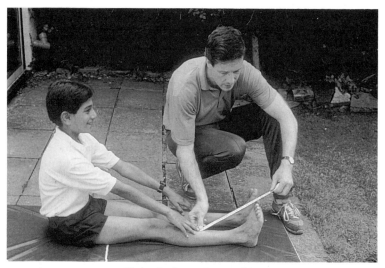

Measuring hamstring stretching.

strings is always done with caution, whether it is part of a flexibility programme or a remedial exercise following injury. The child sits with the injured leg forward and the other leg tucked out of the way. Keeping the back straight and head up, he or she gently leans forwards to bring the chest towards the thigh. If the hamstrings are very tight, the child may have to stretch both legs together, aiming simply to sit up straight with both legs forwards. One treatment technique which a physiotherapist might do to help extreme tightness is to stimulate the vastus medialis muscle electrically (p. 160), with the child sitting with the foot or feet supported on a roll or block. This helps the child to activate the thigh muscles to press the knee fully straight, thereby stretching the back of the thigh.

Parallel with flexibility, the injured hamstrings have to regain strength and co-ordination. Remedial exercises include free exercises, exercises with light ankle weights or weights boots, perhaps progressing to weights machines such as the leg extension and the hamstring curl. Measuring the hamstring muscle function on computerized equipment (such as the Kin Com, Lido or Cybex) can be a valuable guide to progress. These machines can also be used for remedial exercises, if the child is big enough (p. 95). The tests, numbers 10 and 11 on p. 104, are simpler checks.

The inner thigh, groin and hip

The adductor muscles on the inside of the thigh can be injured through violent or blocked kicking movements, or over-stretching, as in sideways splits. While the adductors themselves extend from the pubic bone to the thigh-bone, longer inner thigh muscles stretch from the pelvis to the inner (medial) side of the knee. Pain from inner thigh injuries can extend from the groin to the knee. If it is localized to the groin, the doctor usually checks whether the child might have a hernia (a protrusion where a binding tissue has broken), or referred pain from the hip, pubis or lower back. Injury to the adductor muscles can affect the hip and the lower back, while the longer inner thigh muscles can also cause stress on the inner side of the knee. The inner thigh muscles are specially likely to be injured in teenagers who are doing too much sport, whether they are running too often or too far, playing too much football or tennis, or using weights that are too heavy on a leg press machine. When the teenager's front thigh muscles are worked beyond their limits, the legs automatically turn inwards, in order to make use of the inner thigh muscles for extra strength, and this causes unnatural stresses on these muscles, and the hips as well.

The hip is often affected secondary to inner thigh muscle injury, and conversely hip problems can cause tightness (spasm) in the groin area, which can mimic or accompany tendon and muscle pain. Of all the problems in the weight-bearing joints, hip injuries are probably the easiest to miss or mis-diagnose, because in many cases the child has no pain directly over the hip itself, but complains instead of knee pain. This is one of the reasons why the doctor always checks the child's hips as well as the painful knee(s). Being the major joint linking the leg with the pelvis and therefore the lower back, the hip can undermine the body's mechanics significantly when it is injured. In children, traumatic hip injuries most often involve the bones and growth plates, and should be treated as emergencies.[15] More minor injuries can alter the hip joint's mechanics, and therefore lead to structural problems. The stresses of growth and excessive sport can cause overload on the hips. If the child is overweight, this adds to the burden on the joints. The tendency for the hips to turn inwards when the child is struggling to achieve certain movements alters the pattern of loading between the flank bone (ilium) and the head of the thigh-bone where they form the hip joint. This might damage the cartilage surface of the head of the thigh-bone, or disrupt the bone's growth area.

Some children have 'snapping hips' which click on certain (usually twisting) movements, or when they are walking upstairs. The sound is caused by a ligament or tendon catching on an underlying structure. The condition usually involves *bursitis* (inflammation in one of the natural fluid-filled cysts) over the outer side of the hip area, but it can have any of several different causes. If there is no pain when the snapping sound occurs, the problem is nothing to worry about, although the child should be checked for limitations of hip movement (tests 13–15, p. 105), and these should be corrected, if present, through remedial exercises. If there *is* pain, it should be treated: physiotherapy is usually used in the first instance, but in the worst of cases the child may need surgery to clear away the bursa if it is badly thickened.

In every case of hip, groin or inner thigh muscle injury, full mechanics must be restored to the hip and pelvic region before the child resumes normal sport. The child must be able to turn the hips inwards and outwards, and stretch the legs backwards equally on both sides. Therefore remedial exercises relate to the thigh, pelvis and lower back: similarly, the tests to check whether full function has been restored cover all these areas (test exercises 8–11 and 13–21, p. 103). Swimming using varied strokes is good exercise to improve hip movement, and the older teenager may use resistance machines, as in the Nautilus, David or Norsk systems, to improve the balance between strength and mobility around the hips. The child's posture also has to be corrected. Standing with the bodyweight balanced on one leg, or sitting crookedly or with legs crossed can have a very bad influence on the hip joints, so the child has to be reminded to sit and stand correctly at all times.

The trunk

Posture is also an important factor in helping to prevent injuries to the trunk, including the abdominal and chest muscles in front, and the lower back up to the neck behind. 'Good' posture is not an absolute truth: there are structural variations between individuals, so children cannot be expected to show identical conformity when asked to sit or stand 'up straight'. However, there are postural habits which are identifiable as 'bad', including slouching, standing, sitting and lying crookedly, holding one's head to one side or slightly

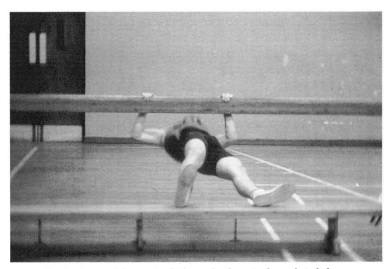

Rowing is one of the sports which can develop spinal muscle imbalance.

twisted, or holding the arms or legs at awkward angles. Bad postural habits in children lead to poor development of the postural muscles. The anti-gravity muscles cannot develop adequate strength and tone if the child spends the greater part of each day hunched over a desk at school or slouched in an easy chair watching television or a computer screen. The more the child is allowed to stand, sit or lie in poor positions, the weaker the postural muscles become, and the less the child is able to correct his or her posture when asked. Poor postural muscles result in joint distortions as the child grows: sitting down all day, for instance, causes stiffness in the ankles, knees, hips and lower back, combined with weakness in all the body's muscles, especially round the shoulders. Awkward sitting creates unbalanced, asymmetical stresses on the joints, especially in the spine.

Many sports also have an effect on the child's posture. Sports which involve applying effort with the trunk bending and twisting tend to create in-built strength and flexibility imbalances in the trunk's controlling muscles. Rowers, for instance, often tend to develop round shoulders: a teenager who learns to row only on one side may also develop a sideways curve in the spine (*scoliosis*). Single-handed tennis players tend to develop a slight sideways curvature, whereas double-handed players may develop hunched, rounded shoulders. A scoliosis can cause an apparent difference in the child's leg lengths, because the pelvis is tilted down on one side. Conversely, a real leg length discrepancy can cause an abnormal pelvic tilt and scoliosis. Either situation might contribute to leg, pelvic or back injuries.[16] A real difference in the measured length of the legs can happen naturally, or it can result from a childhood leg fracture involving a growth plate, where the bone has over-grown or under-grown as it healed.

Trunk injuries can happen to children and teenagers through different mechanisms. The abdominal region is a common site for a 'stitch', which is a painful, cramp-like spasm. The exact cause of the stitch is not known, but it can be linked to exercising too soon after a meal or on an empty stomach. The abdominal muscles and any other soft tissues in the trunk can be injured by similar movements, but the spinal joints tend to suffer the most. The injuries can cause pain in the area of damage, or there may be referred pain (often called a 'trapped nerve'), felt down one or both legs, round the rib cage, or down one or both arms, according to whether the injury has happened in the lower back, middle back or neck. Confusingly, the referred pain may seem just like a muscular ache, and there may not be any spinal pain to indicate its source. In many soft-tissue injuries involving the trunk, the child may also notice similar pain on coughing or sneezing.

In some sports, the need for maximum flexibility in the lower back can lead to excessive stresses in the spinal joints. This is a specific risk in female gymnastics, where it has been found that an exaggerated lordosis can be associated with both reduced spinal mobility and low back problems.[17] The problems are likely to be worse if the girls have stiff shoulders as well as a pronounced lordosis.[18] Repetitive jarring has been found to cause structural damage to the spinal joints in water ski-jumping,[19] and it is possible that similar damage might be associated with horse-riding and motorbike scrambling.

The spine can be overloaded through lifting or throwing excessively heavy weights. In throwing events, children should be carefully monitored when they progress to a heavier implement, while young weightlifters should be restricted to multiple repetition lifts of relatively light weights, and discouraged from any heavy weightlifting until the late teens. Loading pressures can also be sustained from tackles, lifts or throws in contact sports like American football, rugby, judo or wrestling, especially if the opponents are unevenly matched for size, strength and weight. Heading a football can cause over-compression on the child's neck joints.

Even without heavy loading, sharp twisting movements can over-stress the spinal joints, so young squash and badminton players can suffer from back injuries related to over-playing or to a sudden awkward movement. Over-stretching can cause back injuries: forcing toe-touching movements when the legs have lengthened out through the growth spurt can 'pull' the lower back. The middle back (thoracic spine) can be strained if the child lies supine and swings the legs up and backwards to touch the floor behind his or her head. (This Yoga exercise, called 'Halasana', can only be done safely with proper preparation, training and control.) Hard abdominal exercises, such as double-leg-raising lying supine, or excessive sit-ups can increase the pressure in the spinal discs to dangerous levels.

Treatment for trunk injuries in young sports players should always be undertaken with caution. Before any physical treatment starts, the more serious possible diagnoses have to be excluded. The doctor or specialist has to be certain that there is no bone injury, nor any involvement of organs, such as the spleen. If the abdominal muscles are injured, the doctor may check for a hernia. In cases of chest or thoracic pain, the child may have had some illness or infection mimicking or underlying an injury. Once soft-tissue injury is the confirmed diagnosis, treatment may include gentle manipulation or massage techniques by a physiotherapist, osteopath or chiropractor. The younger the child, the less likely the practitioner is to manipulate the spinal joints to any degree. At any age, the child may be given an elastic corset to support the lower back and reduce the disc pressure. It is rare for children and teenagers to suffer major disc damage rather than bone injury, but if it happens, surgery may be needed as a last resort.[20]

In all cases, the trunk and the whole body have to be kept in good alignment through correct, symmetrical posture, and they have to regain full function. Back and abdominal exercises are carefully graded following an injury, so that the child is never doing exercises which revive or aggravate pain. By the end of the rehabilitation period, the child should be able to do all the hip and trunk test exercises freely (p. 107, numbers 17–22). Swimming, using varied strokes, can be useful for combining trunk exercise with aerobic fitness training. Overall body conditioning including specific exercises for the trunk can be achieved on the Norsk Sequence-Training System. If the trunk injury has been directly related to the child's

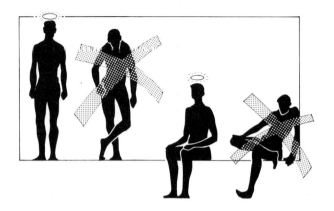

sport, the adults involved have to weigh up carefully whether the child should be allowed to return to that sport. On resuming or taking up any sport after these injuries, the child should be carefully monitored and not allowed to play too much too soon.

The shoulder, arm and hand

The shoulder is the most mobile joint in the body: it is a loose ball-and-socket joint, and forms part of a complex of joints linking the collar-bone (clavicle) to the breast-bone (sternum) and the shoulder blade (scapula). The shoulder blade glides over the ribs in the upper back region, while the collar bone joints (sternoclavicular and acromioclavicular) form more tightly jointed links. There are many growth points in the bones of the shoulder complex, which makes the region especially vulnerable to injuries involving the bones in children and teenagers. However, the shoulder depends purely on its soft tissues for its stability, so these are often injured together with, or separately from, the bones.[21] Shoulder injuries often affect the neck, or are secondary to neck problems or stiffness. They can also cause follow-on injuries lower down the arm in the elbow, wrist or hand.

The shoulder joint complex can be injured through violent stresses, as in athletic throwing events and baseball pitching. In some sports, the shoulder supports the bodyweight as well as being moved through its full range, as in men's and women's gymnastics (especially on the rings and asymmetric bars). The shoulder may be injured by the external force exerted by an opponent in sports like judo, wrestling, American football, rugby, and ice or field hockey. Falls onto the point of the shoulder can damage the acromioclavicular joint. Many sports create muscle imbalance coupled with reduced mobility in the shoulder: a survey of young tennis players, for instance, showed that they had marked limitation of inward rotation, combined with increased outward rotation mobility in their shoulders.[22] Swimmers may over-develop the muscles of the front of the shoulder, relative to the back, if they specialize in front crawl or butterfly, where the back of the shoulder may be over-developed in back-stroke specialists. This type of imbalance can contribute to tendon strains ('swimmer's shoulder'),[23] and 'spontaneous' dislocation or subluxation of the shoulder, backwards if the back of the shoulder is relatively weak, forwards in the case of the back-stroke specialists.

Of all the body's joints, the shoulder is the one most often dislocated or subluxed. The injury is caused by a tear through the joint capsule and ligaments, and is associated with sports like gymnastics, rugby and baseball, besides swimming. It can also happen through falls, for instance while skiing or horse-riding. The most common version is for the head of the arm-bone (humerus) to come out forwards, although it can displace backwards or downwards. You should never try to replace a dislocated shoulder, unless you are confident that you have the necessary training to do so safely. Yanking the arm violently back into place carries a strong risk of damaging the main nerves near the shoulder. It is safer to protect the arm in a sling, and have the casualty taken to the nearest hospital for medical treatment. There is a very high rate of re-injury if the first dislocation happens before the age of 20.[24]

Treatment depends on the severity of the injury: for strains and less serious problems, physiotherapy usually includes remedial exercises, electrical stimulation and perhaps ultrasound, interferential or laser therapy, depending on the age of the patient. For severe recurrent dislocations, surgery may be needed to restore stability to the shoulder. In all cases, the remedial exercises are vital, and they should lead to stability, mobility and co-ordination through the whole shoulder girdle complex, as tested in exercises 22–26 (p. 111).

Elbow problems are associated with throwing events, such as the javelin, and racket games such as tennis. 'Little League Elbow' is the term given to elbow problems among young baseball pitchers, as injuries occur at such a high rate.[25] The growth plates in the bones forming the elbow are complex. Most of the ossification centres at the lower end of the arm-bone are fused by the ages of 15 to 17, but the fusion process can go on until the age of about 20, especially on the outer tips (epicondyles) of the bone, to which the main forearm tendons controlling the wrist and fingers are attached. The head of the radius, the bone on the thumb side of the forearm, fuses at about 17 years, while the elbow end of the ulna, on the little finger side of the forearm, fuses earlier, at 14 to 16 years.[26] Overuse and traumatic elbow injuries in teenagers are therefore likely to affect the bone growth areas, as well as, or instead of, the attached ligaments or tendons. These injuries may take a long time to heal, and perhaps have long-term effects.

Like the shoulder, the elbow can be dislocated by a wrenching force, perhaps in a fall, or an awkward movement in gymnastics, or a rough tackle in American football. Twisting forces can pull the head of the radius out of its containing ligament. Serious elbow injuries carry the risk of extra bone formation (*heterotopic ossification*) resulting in joint stiffness. A direct blow to the elbow can cause myositis ossificans, or bone formation within the arm muscle (brachialis), in the same way as the problem occurs in the front thigh region. More minor injuries include 'golfer's elbow' and 'tennis elbow', which are overuse strains of the tendon insertion points on the inner (little finger) and outer (thumb) sides of the elbow respectively. Both golfer's and tennis elbow are complicated conditions which can involve damage to several different structures.

Serious injuries may require immobilization in a plaster cast, or surgery. Elbow injuries are always treated cautiously: strengthening and mobilizing exercises are never forced, in case the joint is damaged further, or new, unwanted bone growth is stimulated. However, rehabilitation aims to restore full power to the muscles and motion in the joint complex, while maintaining good function in the shoulder above, and the wrist and hand below the injured elbow (test exercises 23–24, 28–30, p. 111). In overuse injuries, the cause has to be identified. If it is linked to inappropriate equipment such as a tennis racket which is too tightly strung, or which has a heavy head, or too wide or too narrow a handle, the child must not be allowed to resume the sport without changing equipment. If the problem was linked to poor technique, for instance in javelin throwing, the coach must teach the child a new, more efficient style. The elbow must recover fully from injury before the child is allowed to resume sports which stress the joint or put it at risk of further injury. If the child returns to sport before the elbow is ready, there is a strong risk of secondary injuries in the shoulder, wrist or hand.

Wrist and hand injuries have increased as more children are doing more sport, and these injuries are particularly associated with trauma from falls or jarring in sports like American football, skateboarding, basketball and skiing.[27] Overuse injuries in the wrist can occur in racket games through over-playing or using inappropriate equipment. The fingers and thumb can be stubbed or wrenched in a variety of situations. A dislocated thumb is often referred to as 'gamekeeper's thumb',[27, 28] but in children, by contrast with adults, the thumb bones are often fractured together with the torn ligaments. The fingers can be dislocated, especially at the main knuckles (metacarpophalangeal joints). If a finger tip is forced backwards, the main tendon which bends the finger can tear, usually breaking off a chip of bone as well. Ball games such as cricket, volleyball and rugby carry the risk of stubbing the fingers, pressing the bones into each other and perhaps causing fractures as well as joint swelling and pain.

Treatment for any hand injury must be accurate, to avoid leaving a permanent impairment in the hand's function, so the child should see the doctor or specialist as quickly as possible after the injury. Fractures, ligament and tendon tears, or bad sprains may need surgery or immobilization in a plaster cast. In less severe injuries the finger might be protected by being taped to its neighbour. After healing, it is vital for the child to regain full co-ordination and balance in the hand and forearm muscles,[29] using detailed exercises including test exercises 27–30 (p. 112). Alongside the movements specific to recovery of hand function, the physiotherapist also prescribes remedial exercises for the rest of the arm and shoulder girdle, to prevent secondary stresses which might cause later injuries.

9 Knee Injuries

The knee is the most commonly injured joint in sports players, and this is especially true among children, as most injury surveys show (see table, p. 77). The knee joint proper, between the thigh- and shin-bones (tibiofemoral joint), is a major weight-bearing joint which is subjected to shearing, jarring and traction stresses during sport. The knee-cap joint with the thigh-bone (patellofemoral joint) is not load-bearing, but it acts as a pulley, guiding the quadriceps muscles and their attached patellar tendon. The knee's mechanics can be distorted by trauma, overuse syndromes or, in the inactive child, insufficient normal movement. If knee problems are not properly treated, the joint itself may suffer permanent damage, leading to early osteoarthritis, and there may be secondary effects of pain or injuries in the thigh muscles, calf muscles, foot, ankle, hip or back.

Knee swelling. A child's swollen knee should always be checked by a doctor or surgeon. If the knee has swollen up for no apparent reason, it might mean that the child has an inflammatory arthritis, or that there is an infection in the joint. The swelling might be painless, but is more likely to be acutely painful. The child may perceive the knee as 'hot', and indeed it may feel hot if you touch it. Occasionally, the knee(s) might swell in this way as a reaction to certain types of food or drink, if they are consumed every day. This type of joint reaction can be associated with spicy foods, chocolate, dairy products like cheese, and acid drinks, particularly orange juice. For an unexplained knee swelling, the family doctor may refer the child to a rheumatologist, who might do blood tests or other checks to find out what is wrong.

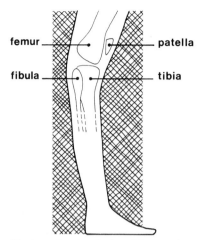

femur — patella

fibula — tibia

The bones forming the knee joint complex.

If the child's knee swells as the result of an injury, such as a jar or a fall, there may be blood or excess synovial fluid (joint lubricating fluid) in the knee, and it should be assessed and treated by a doctor or casualty officer as quickly as possible.[1] They may refer the child to an orthopaedic specialist for diagnosis and, if necessary, surgery. In the first instance, you should treat the swelling immediately with cold compresses or ice packs over a damp towel, held on for between five and fifteen minutes, according to how long the child can tolerate it. You should repeat the treatment at hourly intervals, if there is a delay in getting to the doctor. You can support the knee with a tubular bandage extending about six inches below and above the knee, if this is comfortable to apply, otherwise you can wrap cotton wool wadding round the whole joint and secure it with a crepe bandage.

Cartilage tears. Cartilage injuries can happen to children in much the same way as they do to adults. The soft semilunar cartilages (menisci), which serve as shock absorbers in the knee, can be torn by twisting stresses, for instance when the child turns suddenly and his or her foot sticks in the ground. The damage can happen at any age, but is most common in teenagers who do skateboarding or roller-skating, or play games like football or hockey, especially on artificial surfaces. There may be instant pain and swelling, or the symptoms can come on more gradually. Often, the child seems to recover quickly from the immediate injury, but then develops problems such as locking or giving way, so that the knee does not feel secure under stress when the child is running about or playing games. Sometimes cartilage symptoms develop without any obvious injury, because the child has a congenital malformation of the cartilage known as a *discoid meniscus*.[2] The cartilage is thickened throughout its substance, instead of being thinner in its central part, and so it blocks the knee joint, causing a 'snapping' feeling. When a discoid cartilage is present, it can cause symptoms even before the age of 3: the child might limp, and you may hear an audible click in the knee when the child moves the joint.

If the damaged or discoid cartilage is preventing the knee from functioning properly, the surgeon will probably operate to remove part or all of it. This is technically termed *meniscectomy*,[3] and is usually done through a special probe called an *arthroscope*, if possible, so that the surgeon does not have to cut a scar into the knee. More recently, surgeons have been experimenting with repairing damaged knee cartilages, to help prevent long-term damage to the knee joint surfaces.[4] Physiotherapy to recover full strength and movement in the leg is vital after the operation, and the child should not be allowed to return to sports before rehabilitation is complete.

Cruciate ligament injuries. Like cartilage tears, cruciate ligament strains and tears can happen when the knee is violently bent and twisted, in both adults and children. The ligaments can be injured in very young children, for instance through falls while cycling or skating. In teenagers, awkward movements while changing direction, or violent tackles in sports like rugby, football or hockey, can cause the damage. The two cruciate ligaments bind the centre of the knee joint together, and when they are over-stretched or torn, separately or together, they create instability and a feeling of 'looseness' (technically termed *laxity*) in the knee. The knee might tend to give way or give an audible 'clunk' when it is bent and twisted in a certain way. Occasionally, a loose piece of the torn ligament can make the knee 'lock'. Cruciate ligament injuries often occur together with other damage, such as cartilage tears or bone fractures, and they usually cause swelling. Accurate diagnosis is essential for correct treatment,[5] and this is normally done by the orthopaedic surgeon. It may be necessary for the child to have an operation to stabilize the knee,[3] or the surgeon may recommend physiotherapy, to achieve stability through remedial exercises.[6] Remedial exercises are given for all the knee muscle groups, but in most cases of cruciate ligament damage, the hamstrings are specially important.[7] The child may also need to wear a supportive brace to protect the knee, particularly during active sports.

Medial ligament injuries. The medial ligament on the inner side of the knee can be injured in children of any age, usually by a force which twists the knee or bends it sideways. There may or may not be swelling, and there is tenderness over the ligament, so the child feels pain if the knees touch each other, for instance in bed at night. Doing the splits sideways can cause this injury in both knees, for instance in a fall during skiing. The injury is very likely to happen if the child has slightly stiff hips, and someone is exerting pressure on the child's shoulders to force the splits position, as sometimes happens in karate training. Young footballers should not copy professionals who slide on their knees to celebrate a goal, as this places immense pressure on the medial ligaments. Breast-stroke swimming and squash can cause overuse medial ligament pain in one or both knees. If the medial ligament is completely torn, and the knee is therefore unstable, the orthopaedic surgeon may operate to make it secure.[8] For more minor medial ligament injuries, physiotherapy treatment is usually the norm, and the child has to lay off any sporting activities which aggravate the knee. A supportive brace which keeps the knee straight may be used to protect the knee from harmful stresses. Remedial exercises, perhaps combined with electrical stimulation, are the usual form of treatment, and any electrotherapy modalities which might disrupt bone growth are avoided. Even a slight medial ligament strain can take several months to heal completely.

Dislocation. If the main knee joint dislocates, it is a very serious injury, as all the important holding structures are broken, and there is a strong risk of damage to the major blood vessels and nerves that cross the back of the joint. If you see the child's knee completely distorted after a fall or a violent injury, you should not try to re-align it. You should keep the child as calm and comfortable as possible, and call the emergency services to transfer him or her to hospital immediately. The child should not be given food or drink, as surgery is likely to be necessary. After surgery, there is likely to be a long period of convalescence, coupled with progressive rehabilitation treatment.

Patella alta. This is the technical name for a high knee-cap, that is a knee-cap unusually high in relation to the horizontal line of the main knee joint. The high knee-cap is especially significant if the knee is also shaped with an exaggerated backward curve (hyperextension), called *genu recurvatum.*[2] This may be a hereditary configuration, and it is often associated with flat feet, but disturbance in the growth part of the shin-bone or thigh-bone can cause genu recurvatum accompanied by patella alta. While injury is often an important cause, posture can be a decisive factor, especially as a high knee-cap can be increased during teenage growth spurts.[9] Wearing high heels can press the knees into a fully extended position, so teenage girls should be discouraged from using more than a slight heel, at least until the age of 17–18 when their main growth phases have passed. Intensive flexibility training can lead to exaggerated knee mobility, and it is often the case that young female gymnasts have patella alta combined with genu recurvatum. In young sports players of both sexes, the high knee-cap often seems to accompany relatively under-developed quadriceps muscles, special weakness in the vastus medialis muscles and compensatory over-development in the calf muscles. Usually, both knees show the same contours, but occasionally one knee has the high knee-cap, with or without hyperextension, while the other is normal.

Patella alta and genu recurvatum need not necessarily cause pain or injuries in themselves, but they can contribute to a basic instability in the knee-cap joint and the main knee joint itself. It has been suggested that contact sports should not be allowed for young sportsmen with this shape of knee, because they are so vulnerable to catastrophic knee injuries when put under the type of stress that occurs in tackles and scrummages, for instance, in American football or rugby.[2] Several types of injury at the front of the knee are often associated with patella alta and genu recurvatum, such as fat pad impingement, plica syndrome, patellar tendon damage, knee-cap pain syndromes including chondromalacia patellae, knee-cap subluxation and dislocation, osteochondritis dissecans, and, inside the front of the main knee joint, cartilage compression. All of these conditions, however, can happen to children with normally shaped knees, or variations apart from patella alta and genu recurvatum.

Fat pad impingement. Impingement of the fat pads which lie on either side of the front of the knee, just below the knee-cap, can happen when the child has genu recurvatum, simply because there is not enough space, so the fat pads tend to get pinched between the knee bones when the joint is straightened. The fat pads can also be injured through direct pressure: a fall onto the knees can bruise the fat pads, or they can be damaged through prolonged kneeling or crouching. Twisting the knee awkwardly can cause shearing stresses over the fat pads. One or both of the fat pads can become tender when a child has knee-cap pain. Bruised fat pads usually respond to treatment with ice and gentle massage, perhaps with heparinoid or arnica cream. If the fat pads are sore secondary to another problem, they usually recover when the main problem is solved.

Plica. A plica is an enlarged fold in the synovial (fluid-forming) lining of the knee joint, and it often happens as a result of traumatic injury to the knee. The plica can become caught when the knee is in certain positions, causing localized pain and tenderness, a feeling of locking or snapping in the joint, and sometimes a little swelling. The symptoms may be similar to those of fat pad impingement, or more like those of a cartilage tear. If the problem does not settle with rest from sport, possibly combined with physiotherapy treatment, surgery may be needed to trim the intruding plica. After surgery, it is vital to re-train vastus medialis (p. 160), as the muscle is often badly inhibited.

Patellar tendon injuries. The patellar tendon, which links the tip of the knee-cap to the tibial tubercle, can be damaged through overuse if a child does too much running or football. It can also tear, totally or partially, through trauma, for instance in a blocked tackle, or if the child falls while jumping up. Between the ages of 10 and 17, overuse patellar tendon injuries are often associated with tibial tubercle pain (Osgood-Schlatter's 'disease', p. 128) or damage to the tip of the knee-cap (Sinding-Larsen-Johansson 'disease', p. 128), although the pain is not necessarily worse if the bones are damaged. Growth spurts can contribute to patellar tendon injuries. In girls, the hips widen as puberty approaches, and this alters the angle of pull of the tendon, technically called the 'Q-angle'. In teenage boys who do a lot of bent-knee activities, such as squash, the hamstrings at the back of the knee can become relatively short, causing increased pressure on the patellar tendon when it has to straighten the knee. When the tendon is injured, it is painful under pressure, and hurts

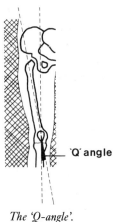

The 'Q-angle'.

when the child walks up and down stairs. If the tendon is torn completely, the knee-cap loses its anchor, so it becomes dislodged onto the front of the thigh. Treatment depends on the severity of the injury: surgery is usually needed for the worst types of patellar tendon problem, but the more common overuse strains generally recover with rest from painful activities, combined with physiotherapy treatment and remedial exercises to create the correct balance of muscles and tendons. A patellar tendon strap can help to relieve the pain in the acute phase.

Knee-cap pain syndrome. Pain from the knee-cap joint is often referred to technically as *retropatellar pain*, and is one of the most common knee problems, especially among teenagers.[4] The child feels pain over the front of the knee when walking up and/or down stairs; crouching and kneeling are painful; the affected knee-cap grates or creaks; it is very painful when pressed down against the thigh-bone, so a firm bandage can make the pain worse; it aches when the child sits still for long periods – this is often called the 'cinema sign'; there may be a sharp pain when the child stands up after sitting; and the knee may tend to 'give way' when the child's full bodyweight is over it, for instance while walking down stairs.

The problem can be triggered simply by the growth phases which alter the mechanics of the knee-cap and the patellar tendon. More commonly, it happens because the child has been doing activities which hold the knees bent, such as playing squash, or field or ice hockey, fencing, skiing, cross-country running, or bicycling with the saddle too low. Because the problem is common in track and distance runners, it is often called 'runner's knee'. Certain exercises can bring on knee-cap pain, especially the popular pre-ski exercise of 'sitting' for long periods against a wall to strengthen the thighs. Sitting still in a chair with the knees bent also interferes with the knee-cap joint's mechanics, so the problem may arise when the child has had long spells watching television, travelling in an aeroplane, or writing school exams. Trauma to the knee-cap, such as a kick, a blow from a hockey stick, or a fall directly onto the knee can also result in the typical pattern of knee-cap pain. If a very young child (below the age of 10) has this type of accident, there may be little pain at the time, although the child might limp. However, the knee-cap can become painful years later, when various factors, including growth, sports activities or inactivity, uncover the basic weakness. Knee-cap pain can occur secondary to other injuries to the main knee joint, such as a twisting injury which damages one of the semilunar cartilages. In the absence of a known injury, the problem can occur as an overuse syndrome in both knees together, or only one. Sometimes the child or teenager experiences pain alternating between each knee over a space of time.

What happens inside the knee-cap (patellofemoral) joint in cases of knee-cap pain is often a mystery. It is relatively common for knee-cap pain to occur without any obvious signs of damage in the joint.[10] This is often confirmed when the orthopaedic surgeon investigates the joint by looking inside it through the arthroscope, only to find no sign of any damage to explain the patient's pain. In some cases, however, the back of the knee-cap or the joint surface on the thigh-bone is visibly damaged. Chondromalacia patellae, which is softening and pitting of the cartilage on the back of the knee-cap, is the most common form of damage in children. However, it is also true that damage such as chondromalacia can be present without necessarily causing pain.

The pain in knee-cap syndromes is due entirely to faulty tracking, which makes the knee-cap 'jar' when the knee is bending under load. The cause of the mal-tracking is poor co-ordination in the vastus medialis muscle, which is the only one of the four quadriceps muscles to control the knee-cap from the inner side. Vastus medialis is inhibited instantly when the knee is injured traumatically, because a protective reflex immediately holds the knee comfortably in a slightly bent position. The muscle loses its normal co-ordination gradually if it is not exercised consistently with knee-straightening movements. It can also be undermined because of normal growth in the leg, especially, for instance, when a teenage girl's hips widen and alter the angle at which the quadriceps and the knee-cap operate.

Therefore, once retropatellar pain syndrome has been diagnosed, and any other possible causes for the child's pain excluded, the treatment regime aims to restore proper co-ordination in the vastus medialis muscle. The practitioner checks whether the knee-cap is being pulled outwards when the quadriceps are tightened with the leg straight, or during squatting movements. Vastus medialis strength is tested with the patient sitting, when the practitioner straightens the patient's leg fully and then asks the patient to hold the knee straight by activating the quadriceps muscles. 'Clarke's sign' is a test which always causes pain: the practitioner blocks the knee-cap movement while the patient tightens the thigh muscles to try to straighten the knee. The back of the knee is checked for tender spots, and the flexibility of the calf, hamstring and quadriceps muscles is tested (pp. 101–4).

Physiotherapists use many different treatment regimes for this condition.[11, 12] This author favours electrical muscle stimulation combined with active knee-straightening exercises to re-educate the

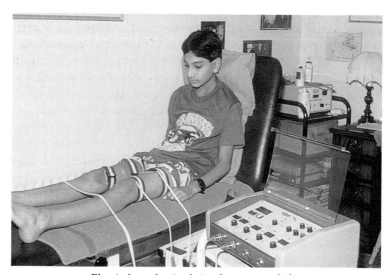

Electrical muscle stimulation for vastus medialis.

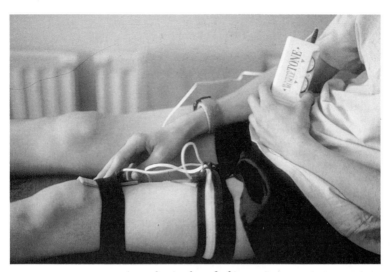

A muscle stimulator for home use.

vastus medialis muscle into co-ordination with the other thigh muscles, in order to improve the knee-cap's alignment during knee movements. For long-standing cases, I teach the child (and/or parents) to use a small muscle stimulator for daily home use. A patellar tendon strap might help to relieve any severe pain. If faulty foot mechanics have contributed to the problem, corrective shoe supports (orthotics) may be fitted by the physiotherapist or podiatrist. The patient is not allowed to do sports which load the bent knee during the recovery process. Advice is given on how to avoid making the pain worse: for instance, the child should not sit still for long periods with the knee bent; walking up and down stairs may be more comfortable done sideways, or one leg at a time.

Remedial exercises include:

1. Twitching the knee-cap by tightening and relaxing the thigh muscles when the knee is straight.
2. Straightening the knee hard while sitting on the floor with a support such as a rolled towel under the heel.
3. Lying on one side and lifting the injured leg straight up sideways.
4. Lying on the stomach and lifting the leg backwards with the knee locked straight.
5. Lying on the stomach with a support under the thigh, to stretch

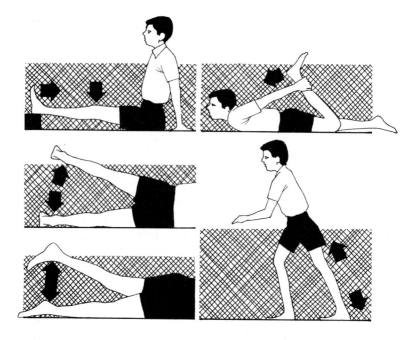

the quadriceps by holding the heel gently towards the seat for a count of ten.

6. Standing with the painful leg behind the other, bending the forward knee, in order to stretch the hind calf gently for a count of ten.

In the later stages of recovery, eccentric quadriceps exercises such as slow knee-bends are added. The straight-leg exercises and the electrical stimulation for vastus medialis are continued until the patient can do squatting movements and normal sports without pain. Even after full recovery, the patient is advised to continue doing some of the straight-leg remedial exercises as a precaution.

If the problem persists, surgery may be needed. It is not usual for the surgeon to scrape the back of the knee-cap nowadays, as this tends to make the knee very painful. The lateral release operation might be used to free the knee-cap, allowing it to track more centrally. Alternatively, the surgeon may choose to re-align the knee-cap by moving the anchor-point of the patellar tendon, in order to improve the knee-cap's movement. Accurate physiotherapy treatment after any of these operations is vital, and it is especially important to re-establish good function in the vastus medialis muscle as quickly as possible.

Knee-cap subluxation and dislocation. If the knee-cap becomes very unstable, either as the result of injury, or simply through a severe loss of muscular control (particularly through vastus medialis), it can be dislodged from its normal position. If it goes out of joint and returns to its place spontaneously, the injury is called *subluxation*; if it remains out of position, it is a *dislocation*. The knee-cap usually subluxes or dislocates outwards (laterally), although occasionally it moves inwards (medially). When the knee-cap dislocates, the knee should be well supported and the child taken to hospital immediately. Very often, the knee-cap can be corrected without difficulty, but the joint remains swollen and painful. After a subluxation or dislocation, a brace or full bandage may be used to hold the knee-cap in its normal position while the child is given physiotherapy treatment and remedial exercises to restore stability. If a child's knee-cap dislocates badly, or more than once, surgery may be needed to repair the joint, followed by physiotherapy to regain co-ordination in vastus medialis and all the other controlling muscles for the knee, using much the same format as the regime for knee-cap pain syndromes.

10 Injury Case Studies

1. A 10-year-old boy was referred by his general practitioner for physiotherapy to his painful knees. He was keen on all sports, including tennis, swimming and cricket, but his main love was soccer. He was in the school team, and his mother described how he was constantly kicking a football about during every spare moment at home.

He had hurt his left knee a year previously, when he went into a slide tackle and was accidentally kicked in the left leg by an opponent. The right knee had started to hurt some four months later, after he had knocked his leg against a wall. Neither knee swelled up at any stage, but the boy felt pain on either side of the knee-cap on certain movements, and the knee-caps seemed to click. The right knee hurt when he ran. He liked to go jogging every day for training, but he could no longer manage this, and he could only limp through half a soccer game at a time because of the pain in both his knees.

The boy's description was not typical of a knee problem: he had no pain going up and down stairs, no ache when he sat still for any length of time, no pain when he stood up after sitting down, and he could kneel down without discomfort. He felt the knee pain when he balanced on one leg and when he squatted down. Both hips were sensitive when they were tested (test exercise 15, p. 107), and he felt the knee pain as each hip was pressed through its full range of passive movement. The left hip was stiffer, and caused more pain than the right.

The boy was given a programme of simple stretching and mobilizing exercises, especially for the left hip. He was allowed to practise kicking a light ball with his left foot (reversing his usual right-footed pattern), although he was kept away from his normal football training with the team. He also had to practise balancing on one leg at a time to improve his hip muscle balance, and to do knee-bending movements within his pain limits, so that he did not lose strength and mobility in his knees. He was allowed to play a little tennis, and encouraged to go swimming as often as possible. Three months later, he was pain-free, and able to re-start his football, with his mother and the team coach taking on the difficult task of persuading him to get back into the game in easy stages.

2. Another 10-year-old boy was referred for physiotherapy for 'flat fleet' because his feet hurt when he ran. His teachers at school had noticed that he ran with difficulty, and his mother became worried when she realized that her son was limping badly and could hardly walk, following an intensive 'School of Sport' week during which he had played hockey and other sports all day, every day.

The soles of the boy's feet had been painful since he was 7. He had first noticed the pain when he went to a school which included a daily sports session in the curriculum. He had not done much sport before this. His feet would hurt on cross-country running, and jumping up to land on his feet would give him sudden sharp pain. He also noticed pain if he sat still for long periods. Wearing different types of shoes did not seem to make any difference to the pain.

The boy's feet were in fact very strong and mobile, with a good arch, and unusually good toe dexterity. His weakness was in his lower leg muscles, which were extremely feeble, especially the right calf. The muscles looked poorly developed and they functioned inefficiently. The boy could not go up and down on his toes at all, even on both legs together, and his balance on each leg was very poor. At nearly 5 feet 2 inches he was tall for his age, and had grown $1\frac{1}{2}$ inches in the previous six months. His mother confirmed that he had been reluctant to stand and walk as a baby, preferring to crawl or drag himself around until he was about 18 months old. She had been worried at the time that when he did walk he looked 'strange' because his ankles seemed to move very stiffly, but her doctor had checked the boy and found nothing wrong.

The boy was given very simple exercises to improve his balance and begin to strengthen his lower legs (test exercises 1–4 and 6, p. 100). Three weeks later, he was already much improved: he could walk on his toes and his one-legged standing balance was better. He was therefore given a more extensive programme of exercises to add to the original movements, including using a wobble board every day as more advanced balance work (p. 136).

Two months later he was able to walk fairly easily on his toes, and he was making progress with his wobble board balance work. He went on another week-long sports course, and managed to run and play soccer and tennis with very little pain. He was very proud that his time for the 800 metres had improved. He had not had time to try the karate previously recommended to improve his balance. The easier exercises were then dropped from the programme, and several overall strengthening and co-ordination exercises were added (numbers 9, 14, 18, 20, p. 104).

With prompting from both his parents, the boy managed to persevere with his exercises for a time. He also bought a carefully chosen pair of trainers, which he found much more comfortable than his previous models. He was still growing fast, reaching 5 feet 7 inches by the age of 11, a year after his physiotherapy sessions. His feet had ceased to be painful, and he was able to try a wider variety of sports, including badminton and volleyball, when he went on his 'School of Sport' holidays. He could run further than ever before, so he could now enjoy taking the family's dog out for long runs.

3. A 14-year-old girl played a variety of games at school, including tennis, netball and rounders, although she was not particularly keen on sports. She had suffered from right knee pain for one year. She was left-handed. There was no obvious cause for the pain, and it had come on slowly, gradually getting worse. Her doctor diagnosed 'growing pains', but when the pain became worse, he referred her to a rheumatological specialist who diagnosed the problem as 'retro-patellar pain' (p. 158) and referred her for physiotherapy treatment. She had all the typical symptoms: her knee ached when she sat still for long periods, and there was a 'catching' pain when she stood up from sitting. The knee ached when she walked or ran, and going up stairs was particularly painful. The pain had been made much worse when she went on her first skiing holiday with her school.

She had very flexible, hyperextending knees, with very weak thigh muscles. The right vastus medialis was especially weak. Her feet were very pronated with flattened inner arches. The girl was treated with two sessions of electrical muscle stimulation for the right vastus medialis muscle, and her parents bought her a small muscle stimulator which she was taught to use for herself. She used the machine occasionally, but did not enjoy it very much. She wore a small patellar tendon strap to take the pressure off the knee-cap (p. 161). She was also given a programme of remedial exercises (p. 161), and instructed to avoid any sports and activities which stressed her right knee.

She continued to use the machine occasionally for a time, and did her exercises now and then. Her parents preferred not to press her to do her exercises, for fear of exaggerating the knee problem in their daughter's mind. The pain continued to occur intermittently, especially if she sat still for long periods, but the problem gradually improved over the following year, to the point that it no longer interfered at all with her normal daily life.

4. A 16-year-old boy who was keen on skiing, swimming, diving and karate had had knee problems since the age of 6. He 'pulled' his left knee first, and then while skiing at the age of 9 he twisted his right knee so badly that it was in a plaster cast for several weeks. He was always the tallest boy in his class, and his mother had monitored his growth: in some years, for instance when he was 8, he had gained as much as 2 inches. At the age of 14, he was 5 feet 8 inches tall, and he began to notice that after a few days on his skiing trips his knees were hurting, and they would not loosen enough to bend properly without gentle exercises.

By the time he was 16, he was 6 feet $1\frac{1}{2}$ inches tall, and his knees were painful to kneel on, they hurt when he ran any distance, and they would ache if he spent long periods standing up. They did not swell up at all. The pain was limiting his sports activities: he had to cut down his karate, and he had problems riding his bicycle. He was referred to an orthopaedic consultant, who diagnosed 'patellar pain syndrome' (p. 158) and offered to perform the lateral release operation to free the knee-caps. The boy's parents were not satisfied, so they consulted a second orthopaedic surgeon who diagnosed 'growing pains' and referred the boy for physiotherapy. He was also seen by an osteopath, who could find nothing wrong with his knees.

The boy had only slight weakness in his vastus medialis muscles. His right knee was 'looser' than the left when it was fully straightened into hyperextension, but, by contrast, the right knee could not bend as well as the left into the squat position. The boy was treated with electrical muscle stimulation for the vastus medialis muscles, and shown the remedial exercises for patellar pain syndrome (p. 161).

A year later, he had grown even taller, and his knees were better, although he had not done his exercises assiduously. He tended to remember them when his knees ached. He avoided kneeling, in case his knees hurt, and found that they ached and clicked over the knee-caps if he ran more than a short distance. His calves were over-developed relative to his thigh muscles: they were nearly an inch thicker at their broadest point than the lower end of the thighs across the vastus medialis muscles. His lower legs were twisted outwards relative to his thighs, which was a further indication of how much he had compensated through them for the weakness in his thighs. The left thigh was slightly more developed than the right, although the boy was right-handed and right-legged.

He was taught to use a small electrical muscle stimulator, so that he could improve his vastus medialis muscles. He was also given more detailed exercises for the thigh muscles, progressing to squatting movements. It was clear that although the knees were not interfering badly with the boy's preferred activities, he needed to work to improve his thigh muscle function, so that his legs would not be too badly unbalanced when he stopped growing.

5. A keen 17-year-old competitive breast-stroke swimmer developed pain at the back of his left knee through weight training. He felt he might have worked too hard on the hamstring curl machine. He rested for a fortnight, and the problem seemed to have gone, but the front of the knee then started to ache when he was swimming. He normally trained six days a week. The ache spread over the knee-cap region, and onto the patellar tendon and the inner side of the knee. It quickly became worse, giving pain when he walked up stairs, so he rested from all weight-training and leg kicking in the pool. After a month he resumed swimming training, starting with light kicking and building up to normal over the space of a week.

After a few weeks' training, he noticed that the left knee felt 'weak', so he started doing crawl and butterfly to vary his training. Over the space of six months, the pain gradually became worse. The knee was hurting when he walked up stairs, and it would click if he went for a run, giving pain afterwards. His coach referred him for physiotherapy. By this time, he had clear signs of patellar pain syndrome (p. 158), his left knee was very stiff on all movements, and his left hip was also sensitive. Some movements of the hip reproduced the knee pain. He was treated with electrical stimulation to improve the vastus medialis muscle, and given remedial exercises for the thigh muscles and the hip. He maintained his exercise programme religiously, and was pain-free within six weeks of his treatment session.

Eight months later, he had grown about an inch, and he was playing badminton when he turned to the left, balancing on his right leg, and his right knee-cap dislocated. He had not been doing much sport during the preceding three weeks, owing to pressure of exams. On the day of the injury he had been sitting all day in classes, then he did some trampolining for fun, followed by the badminton session. When the knee-cap dislocated, the school matron manipulated it back into place, and the boy was taken to the local hospital casualty department, where the knee was put into a plaster cast. After a month, the plaster was removed, and the boy attended 'knee classes' at the local physiotherapy department three times a week.

The knee was gradually gaining stability as the thigh muscles became stronger, but it still felt weak when he walked up stairs. When he squatted down the knee-cap still pulled badly outwards, and caused pain. The boy was treated with electrical stimulation for the vastus medialis muscle, and taught to use a small muscle stimulator for home exercise. He worked at his home programme until he was pain-free, and then gradually returned to sport. By this time, he had stopped serious swimming training to concentrate on his examinations, but he was hoping to resume competitive sport when he reached university.

6. A 13-year-old competitive gymnast hurt her back one day during a tumbling session. She was in severe pain, but after a couple of days, she tried to continue her normal training, leaving out backward movements and 'walkovers'. She normally trained on four days a week for about three hours at a time. After two weeks, her pain became severe: she was in pain if she sat down, although this eased slightly if she lay backwards against a support; her back hurt when she walked, stood still, or balanced on her left leg; she also had difficulty sleeping at night because of the pain.

A month after the original injury, the girl was in acute pain, and had to stop all gymnastics training and sport. Her gymnastics coach referred her for physiotherapy. The girl had a small, thin build, although she had grown about an inch during the previous year. Her pain spread from the left hip region across the lower back. She had a very pronounced lordosis. There was acute tenderness on gentle pressure over the whole pelvic area, extending up to the twelfth rib on the left side. When the girl moved in any direction standing up, she felt immediate back pain: she could hardly bend forward at all. Her left hip was also sensitive on pressure (test 15, p. 107), and the hip was turned inwards relative to the right side.

Because of the severity of the pain, the girl was recommended to lie down in bed for a few days, to see if the acute phase would subside. She did this, taking warm baths at intervals, and using ice over the lower back to ease the pain. After four days, she felt slightly better, and began to get up for short spells each day. She then felt well enough to go back to school, but soon experienced back and leg pain through sitting down for long periods. One day she was sitting in an armchair, but as she stood up, she fell over, and found she could not walk. She lay down, feeling dizzy, and then managed to get up and take a few steps, although her back was hurting badly.

She was referred immediately to a consultant rheumatologist, who diagnosed that she probably had a spondylolisthesis (p. 124). He did not want to confirm this with X-rays, because of the risk of harming the girl. He also felt that a bone scan might not be helpful because the normal epiphyseal changes in the bones would make it difficult to interpret accurately. He therefore strongly advised the girl and her parents that she should give up gymnastics, at least for the foreseeable future. She was to have a long period of rest from sport, coupled with a very careful programme of strengthening exercises for her trunk and limbs. She had to accept, reluctantly, that her competitive gymnastics career was at an end.

7. A 15-year-old competitive tennis player was suffering from right elbow pain. The pain came on gradually as he began to play more intensively when the tournament season started. He was playing two or three matches each day, and noticed the pain after the first tournament, but tried to ignore it and play on. He had used the same racket for about two years, and it was re-strung regularly to the same tension. His father was also his tennis coach, and he took particular care in choosing appropriate equipment for his son. As the elbow pain became worse, the boy started to rest instead of playing on Sundays, but after four weeks the pain was so bad he had to stop altogether. It had only affected his service at first, but then he found

it painful on both forehand and backhand.

The boy was treated by a physiotherapist at his tennis club, who referred him to a consultant orthopaedic surgeon. X-rays were taken, an overuse syndrome diagnosed, and the arm was protected in a sling. A second orthopaedic surgeon was consulted, and he referred the boy to a hand specialist for nerve conduction tests, because he noticed that the boy's hand was weak and he could not feel sensations normally. The tests were normal, so the boy was referred to a consultant rheumatologist, who took further X-rays and then referred him for physiotherapy.

At this stage, seven months after the problem started, the boy was unable to practise tennis for more than ten minutes without feeling the elbow pain. If he played any longer, the pain would last for several hours. The elbow tended to 'lock' at least once a day, and would only straighten out again if the boy clicked it free, which was painful. It hurt sometimes on normal activities such as eating, and was particularly painful if he played darts. There was tenderness on pressure on the tip of the elbow, and over the heads of both forearm bones. The common flexor tendon on the inner side of the elbow was tender to touch and painful on movement ('golfer's elbow'). The elbow was held slightly bent, and could not straighten fully. The boy was quite tall: he had grown during the year, and he had a strong, muscular build.

He was given a simple programme of stretching exercises for all the elbow muscle groups, instructed to use ice or hot-and-cold dips every day, and told to avoid all games involving the arm. Six weeks later, he was much better: the elbow was 'locking' less often, and the pain was reduced. However, there was now localized pain at the back of the elbow, especially when the joint was straightened suddenly. It was also clear that the boy's hand was contributing to his elbow problems. He had had problems writing his exams, completing them with his left hand, and he was unable to grip objects if his arm was held straight with the palm facing upwards. The inner side of his palm, his little finger and his index finger were very weak. It then transpired that the boy had broken his fifth finger six months before the elbow problem had started, and had knocked the hand again while his arm was in a sling to protect the elbow.

The next part of the remedial programme included specific exercises for the fingers and the palm of his hand, coupled with two sessions of electrical stimulation for these muscles. The boy also started training on the Norsk Sequence-Training equipment (p. 27) to improve his overall condition. Within six weeks, twelve weeks after starting the rehabilitation programme, his pain had resolved, and he was able to perform all the normal hand and arm movements without any problems. He resumed tennis, and played in the summer tournaments. He gained an inch in height, and then started to feel right shoulder pain from serving practice. This seemed to resolve following a treatment session of massage and gentle manipulations (mobilizations), but ten days later he developed middle back pain, again associated with serving. He was treated with mobilizations and electrical muscle stimulation, given remedial exercises, and encouraged to resume his Norsk training, especially to improve his posture.

The middle back region continued to niggle throughout the winter, preventing the boy from doing exercises like press-ups and sit-ups. In the spring, his lower back 'gave' as he served, giving him such acute pain that he could not stand up. He had grown again, reaching 5 feet 10 inches at the age of 16, and he was looking thinner than before. His back was treated with ice and mobilizations, and he was reminded to revive his remedial exercises. He was due to go abroad to start his career as a professional tennis player, and it was clear that he would have to concentrate on protective exercises if he was going to be fit enough to cope.

8. A 17-year-old competitive gymnast was the middle person in a sports acrobatics trio. The trio had been practising together for one month when the girl began to experience back pain. She felt it was related to balance work rather than catching, as the top girl was very light. She first felt pain immediately after training sessions, and it would last until the following day. Resting from training made the back better, so she had a month off. However, on re-starting, it was getting progressively worse as she tried to build up into her normal balance work supporting the top girl. She had tried having osteopathic manipulation after her training sessions, but although this eased the pain at the time, it was not preventing it from recurring.

Her gymnastics coach referred the girl for physiotherapy. She was a slim, slight build. Her back hurt when she bent sideways and backwards, although she could bend forwards without pain. Her right hip was turned out relative to the left, and it was sensitive on pressure tests. She was noticeably weak on the left side when her side-trunk strength was tested (test 18, p. 108). She was treated with very gentle mobilization techniques for the right hip and lower back, given a series of strengthening exercises for all the trunk muscle groups, and advised about maintaining correct posture. After this, she attended training sessions using the Norsk Sequence-Training equipment.

She was much better, and continued her normal training without problems for three months. However, the training increased in preparation for a championship, and her back pain recurred after a particularly heavy routine of catching. The pain spread over both hips and the lower back. The right hip felt very stiff, and gave a 'click' on certain movements. All her back movements were restricted, so she was treated again with gentle mobilization techniques for the lower back and both hips, and given careful remedial exercises. She managed to compete in the championships ten days later, but gave up gymnastics soon afterwards, partly because of her back problems, and partly for other interests.

Two years later, the girl took up dancing and aerobics. She was all right for a couple of months, managing to exercise on four days a week, but then she started to feel twinges in her left hip when she landed from jumping. There was some reaction in the right hip as well, but it was the left leg which gave way one day when she landed from a high leap. She had severe pain the next day, extending from the hip region down the inner thigh. When she attended for physiotherapy, her left quadriceps muscles were relatively tight (test 8, p. 103); her right hamstrings were stiff; her left hip was turned inwards, and it gave a click on stress testing (test 15, p. 107); she was still weak on the left side of the trunk. She was treated again, and given remedial exercises to try to correct her muscle imbalance, after which she managed to return to dancing without problems for nearly a year.

At the age of 21, she took up work as a waitress, which involved long hours and heavy lifting. She developed an acute right-sided back pain one night, which coincided with the onset of her period. It remained acute for several days, so the girl was referred to a consultant rheumatologist who admitted her to hospital and took blood tests and X-rays. She remained in hospital for several days, and within two weeks her back felt almost normal, although not perfect. Her neck had been aching, and she had developed a bad sore throat, so she rested for several more days. She was fitted with

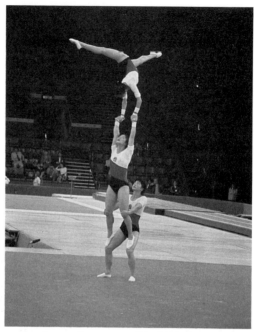

Sports acrobats have to be strong, agile and lightweight, in combination.

an elastic support corset to wear in case of future episodes of acute back pain. She then went to work abroad for six months, where she had no further problems, even though her job involved heavy lifting.

On her return home, she had another episode of acute right-sided back pain, extending up to the right shoulder-blade and down to the right hip. She had felt run-down, as though she had 'flu, during the previous week. Over the next week her neck glands became swollen and she had bad headaches. The rheumatologist saw her again, and felt that, as the girl's brother was suffering from an inflammatory arthritis, she might have a similar problem, even though her blood tests did not show it. He therefore recommended her to rest during the acute pain episode, but to resume protective exercises as soon as she felt able to do so. She had to improve her diet, and she was advised to take vitamin supplements. This was likely to be the pattern of self-care she would have to follow for the foreseeable future.

11 Diet for Children

By Jane Griffin

A healthy balanced diet is essential for everyone, but especially for children. It must provide all the energy and nutrients that are needed for growth and development. Any form of activity, from running around in the playground to training in a particular sport, will place further demands on these requirements. In addition, good dietary habits learnt when young often persist throughout life. These habits are more likely to come from the example of other people (parents particularly) than from any form of health education. A healthy diet means a healthy child, which in turn means a healthy adult.

Much has been reported and written about the state of the British Nation's diet and recommendations to change it abound. Faulty nutrition in childhood has been blamed by many doctors and nutritionists as a cause of disease in later life. Children may 'enjoy' poor eating habits such as excessive intakes of fat, salt and sugar, and these are carried into adult life. Alternatively heart disease, high blood pressure and obesity may be a *direct* result of unhealthy food intakes in childhood. This is a topic of considerable controversy and as yet many questions remain unanswered. Parents may be attempting to adopt healthier eating habits and may wish their children to do the same. However, children are not small adults. What is sensible for grown-ups may be harmful for young children. For instance, a diet low in fat and high in fibre can result in poor weight gain and loose stools in a toddler. When feeding children one needs to keep things in perspective. For instance, diet is not the only cause of heart disease (preventing your child from taking up smoking should be a major consideration) and there is no clear evidence to support the idea that giving babies and small children very sweet food will mean that they will prefer such food for evermore. Too much inappropriate sugar will increase the risk of tooth decay, however, and for that reason the habit should be discouraged.

The importance of a balanced diet

The diet must provide sufficient nutrients for growth, body repair and all the child's activities. The meals must also be liked by the child. No matter how full of nutrients the meal is, it is worth nothing if it is not eaten. Let us look briefly at some of the main nutrients in a child's diet. More detail will be given in the relevant sections further on in the chapter.

Energy. Children have a high energy or calorie intake in relation to their bodyweight, but there is often a limit to the actual amount of food they can eat. It is important to provide foods that are full of nutrients as well as calories. They should not be given cakes, biscuits and sugary drinks in preference to other foods, as these items tend to be high in calories but low in essential nutrients, i.e. supplying energy but little in the way of vitamins, minerals or protein. Most children are good at getting enough to satisfy their energy needs for growth, but it is important that they are offered nutritious foods.

Protein. This nutrient is found mostly in milk products, meat and

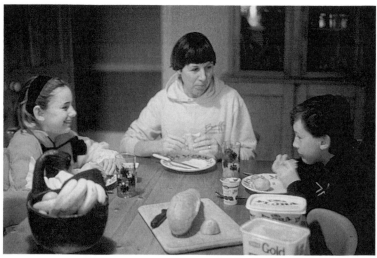

A balanced diet is essential for healthy growth.

cereals, and it provides the material for growth and repair of the body.

Fat. Fat makes food tasty as well as providing energy, essential fatty acids and fat-soluble vitamins. Although it would do most adults good to eat less fat, cutting back a child's intake too drastically can lead to a shortage of energy and essential nutrients.

Fibre. It is not known how much fibre babies and children need, but foods containing fibre should be given where there is a choice. For instance, fibre can be introduced naturally into the diet by offering wholegrain breakfast cereals, wholemeal or white soft-grain bread and fresh fruit and vegetables. Bran and bran-enriched products are not recommended for babies and children.

Minerals. Amongst the fifteen or so minerals that are essential to the human body, there are two that are particularly important for growing children. Calcium is needed for bone and tooth formation, and an adequate intake is vital during periods of rapid growth. Iron is needed for healthy blood.

There are many more different essential nutrients that a balanced diet needs to contain including a whole range of vitamins, minerals and trace elements. But although children need nutrients, they eat food. To help plan a balanced diet, food can be divided up into four main groups. Eating a good variety of foods from these basic groups ensures that children receive all the essential nutrients they need. The groups are set out below.

Basic Food Groups

Group One	**Cereal foods and starchy vegetables:** Bread, flour, oats, rice, corn, breakfast cereals, pasta, potatoes. **Provides**: Energy, fibre, protein, vitamins, minerals. Little fat.
Group Two	**Fruit and vegetables:** Fresh, raw and cooked – all types. **Provides:** Vitamins C and A, folic acid, calcium, iron. Little fat.

Group Three	**Meat and alternatives:** Meat, poultry, fish, pulses (beans, peas, lentils), eggs, nuts. **Provides:** Protein, vitamins, minerals, energy. Fibre from pulses. Fat from meat and meat products.
Group Four	**Milk and milk products:** Milk, cheese, yoghurts. **Provides:** Protein, some vitamins, energy, fat, calcium, phosphorus.

There are two other food groups which increase the energy content of the diet but do little else, and they should not play a large part in the daily diet of most children:

Group Five	**Sugar, sugary foods and drinks:** Sugar, sweets, chocolate, honey, jams and marmalades, sweet biscuits, cakes, jellies, sugary drinks. **Provides:** Energy.
Group Six	**Fats and oils:** Butter, margarine, vegetable oils, lard, suet, cream, salad cream, mayonnaise. **Provides:** Energy, fat soluble vitamins, essential fatty acids.

Pre-school children

After their first birthday, children can usually start to share in the family meal and eat most of the dishes that are prepared for the more grown-up members of the family. Sometimes minor changes are needed so that they can enjoy and cope with the food according to their level of development. Children are changing individuals and the developments which take place between 1 and 5 years of age are enormous and directly and indirectly affect eating habits.

At this stage, children are totally dependent on others for their food. The eating habits and likes and dislikes of their parents and other carers will be those that they imitate and acquire. They should be offered a wide variety of foods with different tastes, textures and colours to help keep their interest. Foods from other cultures can be given as well.

Children are not designed to eat large amounts of food at

infrequent intervals, as they have relatively small stomachs and often small appetites. The typical adult pattern of two or three meals a day and no snacks is not necessarily right for toddlers. Such a pattern can lead to hunger, bad temper and belligerent demands for biscuits, crisps and sweets. Offering a regular pattern of three small meals and two or three nutritious snacks is much better from a nutritional point of view. (The atmosphere will no doubt improve too!)

Appetite is normally a sound guide to requirements, as eating at this age is far less a matter of habit than it is for adults. It is common *and natural* for young children to eat voraciously for one or two days and then to lose all interest in food. Children, like adults, do have days when they don't feel hungry or want to eat a particular food and, unlike adults, children tend to have no choice in what they are given to eat. There is no need either to restrict meals or to force feed on these days.

Energy requirements for children vary enormously, especially as the level of their physical activity varies so much. Tables of Recommended Daily Amounts (RDA) of food energy and nutrients are published by the Department of Health and Social Security,[1] but these are of more use to people supplying food to large groups of people rather than to individuals or families. The best guide that food intake is satisfactory is to carry out three-monthly checks on height and weight and to record the results on a percentile growth chart.

In 1984 the Committee on Medical Aspects of Food Policy (COMA) produced a report entitled *Diet and Cardiovascular Disease*.[2] Its recommendations were to reduce total fat intake to no more than 35 per cent of the total energy of the diet, to avoid obesity; to increase the fibre content of the diet; and to prevent any further increase in salt intake. Although its recommendations are not applicable to children under 5 years of age, there should be a *very* gradual introduction to a healthy COMA-style diet from weaning, so that the recommendations are achieved by around the age of 5. This can be done by following these practical suggestions.

1. Excessive intakes of fat should be avoided by using leaner cuts of meat, trimming off any visible fat, serving poultry (without skin) and fish more frequently, avoiding fried foods by using the grill rather than the frying pan, giving crisps and chips on a less regular basis.

2. The fibre content of the diet should come from that naturally

present in foods, e.g. wholemeal bread, wholegrain cereals, oats, wholewheat pasta, vegetables (especially beans and peas), fruit and nuts.

3. The taste for salt is an acquired one, and good habits in childhood lead to better habits in later life. Salt can be kept to sensible limits by restricting the amount used in cooking and by not putting the salt-cellar on the table. Herbs and spices can be used as salt substitutes to enhance the natural flavour of many foods.

4. Excessive sugar in the diet can spoil the appetite and push out the more nutritious foods. It is also a major factor in tooth decay. Sugary foods and drinks should not form the major part of the diet. Being too strict, however, about sweets etc., can cause problems later on when the child becomes more independent. A compromise, such as sweets once a week, *after* a meal, followed by a good tooth-cleaning session may be the solution.

5. Snacks ensure there is no short-fall in energy intake, but they can lead to uncontrolled intakes of energy too. Suitable nutritious snacks for this age-group include: milk; fresh fruit; wholemeal bread or toast; sandwiches of peanut butter, pure fruit spread, mashed bananas, lean cold meat, cottage cheese, salad vegetables and canned fish; wholegrain breakfast cereals with milk; yoghurt; and muesli bars.

6. Water is an essential element in the body and children should be encouraged to drink some plain water every day as well as unsweetened fruit juice and milk.

There is considerable confusion about which type of milk is best for a pre-school child. In 1989 the Committee on Medical Aspects of Food Policy (COMA) produced a report entitled *Present Day Practice in Infant Feeding*.[3] It recommends that whole cow's milk should be used until at least 5 years of age. Skimmed milk and semi-skimmed milks are not recommended because of their low energy density and vitamin A content. Where semi-skimmed milk is in general use in the home it can be gradually introduced into a child's diet from the age of 2 years, as long as sufficient energy and fat-soluble vitamins are obtained from other sources. It is strongly recommended that fully skimmed milk should *not* be given below the age of 5 years.

Many children dislike particular foods without ever tasting them. They often have a limited range of favourite foods which are constantly being repeated in the daily diet. The chances of having a well-balanced diet are much greater the more variety there is: aim to offer a range of foods from each basic food group over the week. Here is a sample menu.

Sample Menu for a Pre-School Child

On waking	Fruit juice (unsweetened).
Breakfast	Wholegrain cereal – porridge, Weetabix, etc. – with whole milk.
	Wholemeal bread or toast with butter or margarine high in polyunsaturated fatty acids (PUFAs); honey, marmalade, jam, peanut butter or yeast extract.
	Whole milk to drink.
	Vitamin supplement and fluoride tablet or drops.
Mid-morning	Whole milk or unsweetened fruit juice to drink.
	Piece of fruit.
Midday	Minced or chopped meat dish, flaked fish or a vegetarian meal including pulses.
	Chopped or mashed potato, pasta or rice.
	Chopped or mashed vegetables.
	Fruit, ice-cream, custard, yoghurt or milk pudding.
	Whole milk to drink.
Tea	Well-cooked egg, baked beans, cheese, liver sausage, peanut butter.
	Wholemeal bread and butter or margarine high in PUFAs.
	Fruit or yoghurt.
	Water to drink.
Bedtime	Whole milk to drink.

The requirements for vitamins are relatively increased in childhood, and vitamin supplementation is recommended for babies and young children from 5 months up to at least 2 years and preferably 5 years. A daily dose of approximately:

vitamin A	200 µg
vitamin C	20 mg
vitamin D	7 µg

is recommended in the United Kingdom.

'Toddler won't eat' syndrome. Phases of different eating patterns are common in the pre-school years and they can take the form of:
1. Eating very little of anything.
2. Eating well from a very narrow range of foods.
3. Eating a bizarre combination of foods (to an adult's taste).
4. Sudden likes and dislikes.
5. Demanding a particular pattern of eating for security.
These problems are common and don't usually last long – even though it feels like it. No lasting harm results from this behaviour and as long as the child is fit and active, there is no need to worry. Eating problems should never become an 'issue' as it is then so easy to turn mealtimes into battle-grounds: having a relaxed attitude may just help the phase pass more quickly as well.

Weight control. A fat child is not necessarily a happy child. The incidence of obesity in Western children is increasing due to poor dietary habits and lack of exercise. Many parents assume that a fat child will grow out of it but, unfortunately, this is not always the case. However, changes to the diet at this age to control weight should be carried out under the guidance of a doctor and possibly a dietician as well. It should be remembered that as the pre-school child is totally dependent on others for its food, obesity is entirely the fault of the carers and not the child.

Hyperactivity. Although, as the term implies, hyperactive children are constantly on the move, their clumsiness and poor co-ordination make taking part in any organized form of physical activity difficult. A child who is hyperactive leaves one in no doubt that he or she has a behavioural problem, and should not be confused with a child who is just naturally over-boisterous. For this reason, you should never make changes to the diet until a medical diagnosis has been made.

A hyperactive child usually sleeps very little, fidgets a lot and has a short attention span. Aggressive behaviour makes him or her extremely anti-social, and the child will often be labelled troublesome, naughty and difficult in school. Another hallmark of hyperactivity in children is clumsiness. He or she will collide with things, making such activities as cycling and swimming hazardous. Co-ordination is poor and difficulty may be experienced doing up buttons, zips or shoelaces. As he or she gets older, other physical problems such as hay fever, asthma, headaches and abdominal complaints may be experienced.

The cause of hyperactivity is still disputed, but diet seems to play an important part and dietary manipulation has proved successful in many cases. The diet is based on the work of an American doctor, Ben Feingold. He looked at the effect some foods and food additives had on behaviour and learning ability in children. In his diet, all food and drink containing artificial colours and flavours, glutamates (including monosodium glutamate), nitrites and nitrates, butylated hydroxyanisole (BHA), butylated hydroxytoluene (BHT) and benzoic acid are eliminated from the diet. Initially foods containing natural salicylates (aspirin-like compounds) (see the table below) are avoided for four to six weeks, then gradually introduced one at a time to identify any that cause hyperactive reactions.

While hyperactivity remains controversial amongst the medical profession (some doctors denying its very existence), many parents of children with behavioural problems have found that dietary intervention has been helpful. Great care is needed to ensure that the diet remains balanced and provides all the energy and essential nutrients that a growing and active child needs. It is therefore important to find a doctor who is sympathetic, and if your own is not, the self-help Hyperactive Children's Support Group may be able to advise (see Useful Addresses, p. 209).

Natural Salicylates

Fruit	Apples, apricots, cherries, dried fruit, gooseberries, grapes, melon, nectarines, oranges, plums, pineapple, prunes, rhubarb, most berries.
Vegetables	Carrots, cucumber, onion, peas, tomatoes.
Cereals	Maize.
Nuts	All, especially peanuts and almonds.
Beverages	Tea, coffee.

Food intolerance

Food intolerance is an unpleasant or adverse reaction to a specific food or food ingredient which happens every time that food item is eaten, even when the food is given 'blind', i.e. the child doesn't know it is being given. Food allergy is a form of food intolerance, involving the body's immune system. Most cases of food intolerance, including sensitivity to food additives, are not true allergic reactions. Though the reactions may be the same, the immune system is not involved.

The foods most commonly associated with food intolerance are cow's milk, eggs, cereals (especially wheat), tomatoes, citrus fruit, fish (especially shellfish), pork, bacon, chocolate, coffee, tea, preservatives and colouring. Diagnosis of food intolerance is not easy: testing foods under the tongue, checking the pulse rate after ingestion of suspect food, and hair analysis are all unreliable methods and have little use in clinical practice. The ideal is a dietary investigation, carried out under the supervision of a qualified dietician. Sometimes the diagnosis is straightforward. A record is kept of the foods eaten and the appearance of symptoms. This is particularly effective when symptoms appear at once and can be linked with the food just eaten. When symptoms appear later, the cause is often less apparent. Such symptoms include abdominal pain, vomiting, diarrhoea and flatulence, nettle rash and eczema, runny nose, hay fever and asthma, and headache and migraine. In this case diagnosis is by trial exclusion. The child is started on a very strict diet (avoiding all the foods that commonly cause reactions) and gradually foods are introduced back into the diet. Any food which sets up a reaction is then withdrawn again.

Once the diagnosis has been made and the offending foods identified, a process which can take weeks if not months, those foods or food ingredients are removed from the diet. This includes all manufactured foods that contain the items to be avoided. The foods that have to be avoided may make significant contributions to the nutrient intake of a young child, e.g. milk, and the help of a dietician will be needed to devise a diet avoiding the offending foods but at the same time ensuring that the energy and nutrient requirements are being met, particularly if that child leads a physically active life and therefore has an increased energy requirement.

If a food intolerance is suspected, it is vital that the diagnosis and eventual treatment are carried out only under the supervision of a qualified dietician, preferably in an allergy clinic.

School-age children

The general principles outlined already apply to healthy school-age children. Their eating patterns and taste preferences will have been established by the family eating habits during the pre-school years. Any poor habits acquired will be difficult to change. Children like familiar foods and concepts of long-term health tend to cut no ice with them. School-age children have more freedom about what they eat than their younger brothers and sisters. Many forage for snacks themselves, some choose their own school meal, some even have to get their own meals, such as breakfast or a substantial snack after school.

Breakfast. Breakfast seems to be the most frequently missed meal of the day. Children are too keen on the extra time in bed and then have to rush off to school. Breakfast is often not a family meal, with parents setting a bad example by going to work without breakfast. A child who misses this meal may go as much as eighteen hours without food, which is far too long for a growing child. Children who miss breakfast tend to lack concentration during the morning and complain of tiredness and headaches. They may also compensate by eating too many sugary, fatty snacks during the morning. Breakfast should always be eaten, even if it is only a drink and a slice of toast.

The school meal. The midday meal is not just a stop-gap between breakfast and the evening meal, and children should be guided in their choice of food at it. It is important to be aware of the type of meal and foods offered and eaten at midday. Since the 1980 Education Act, Local Education Authorities in the United Kingdom are no longer obliged by law to provide meals for the majority of children, although in fact most do. However, those school meals that are provided do not have to meet any nutritional standards as these were also abolished by the 1980 Education Act. If the school does not provide a satisfactory meal, the alternative is to send the child with a nutritious packed meal. When planning a packed meal, bear in mind that there is often insufficient time in the lunch break for the youngest and the slow eaters to consume very much. To help keep such a child's interest offer small amounts of several items rather than just a pile of sandwiches and a drink.

Evening meal. This is the meal when the day's intake can be balanced up. For instance, if lunch has been rather short on fresh vegetables, a good portion can be served now. Similarly, fresh fruit should be served if the lunch-time meal contained a milk pudding or yoghurt. By using the Basic Four Food Groups (p. 177), the day's intake can be balanced up so that a wide variety of foods from each group is offered. For many children, the evening meal cannot be a family meal because the grown-ups eat too late. As a rule of thumb, if the evening meal is later than 7 o'clock, children under the age of 10 will need to have a separate meal.

Snacks. Active children burn up a lot of energy and with their high nutrient requirements for growth and physical activity, snacks feature quite prominently in the diet of most school-children. Ideal snack items include bread, sandwiches, rolls, wholegrain breakfast cereals, fruit (fresh and dried), yoghurt, milk and milkshakes, cheese, nuts and eggs. Frequent consumption of snacks may cause a loss of appetite at mealtimes, which in turn can lead to a poor nutrient intake, if the snacks are not of a nutritious nature. Here is a sample menu for normal nutrition for school-children:

Sample Menu for a School-child

Breakfast	Unsweetened fruit juice.
	Wholegrain cereal including muesli with semi-skimmed milk or low fat yoghurt.
	Wholemeal bread or toast; butter or margarine high in PUFAs; honey, marmalade, jam, yeast extract.
	Extras – egg, grilled bacon, baked beans.
	Tea, coffee, cocoa.
Midday	School meal, or:
	Wholemeal bread or rolls; butter or margarine high in PUFAs; assorted fillings – cheese, lean meat, egg, fish, peanut butter etc.
	Salad or raw vegetables.
	Fruit, dried fruit, yoghurt, nuts or cheese.
	Water or fruit juice.
After-school snack	Sandwich, fruit and glass of milk.
Evening meal	Meat, fish, pulses.
	Potato, pasta, rice or wholemeal bread.
	Vegetables or salad.
	Fruit, yoghurt, ice-cream or pudding.
	Milk or cheese to finish the meal.
	Drink of milk, water or fruit juice.

Bedtime	Drink of milk, tea, coffee or cocoa.
	Bowl of cereal or sandwich for hungry older
	children.

Weight control. Childhood obesity should not go unchecked, though prevention is, of course, better than cure. Dramatic weight loss is not desirable in children. In general, it is better if a child 'holds' or 'grows into' his weight. During this period of weight-holding, it is important that a healthy, varied diet is still offered. If the child is more than mildly overweight, the advice of a doctor and/or dietician should be sought. The overweight child should not be made to feel different from other children and it may help for the whole family to look at their lifestyle and eating habits and to make modifications. As well as benefiting the family's health, such measures may also help to prevent other members of the family from becoming overweight. All members of the family should be encouraged to:

1. Not add sugar to drinks and cereals.
2. Choose a wholegrain breakfast cereal which does not contain added sugar.
3. Use wholemeal bread and pasta, and brown rice.
4. Eat more fresh fruit and vegetables.
5. Limit chip intake to only once a week – eating more jacket or baked potatoes.
6. Eat fewer cakes, biscuits, puddings, sweets and chocolate.
7. Use low calorie squashes, unsweetened fruit juices or water.
8. Avoid fried foods.
9. Eat only at mealtimes and 'recognized' snack times, e.g., for school-children, when they get home in the afternoon.

Teenagers

'Teenagers are not fed; they eat. For the first time in their lives they assume responsibility for their own food intakes. At the same time they are intensely involved in day-to-day life with their peers and preparation for their future lives as adults. Social pressures thrust choices at them, to drink or not drink, to smoke or not to smoke, to develop their bodies to meet sometimes extreme ideals of slimness or athletic prowess. Few become interested in food and nutrition except as part of a cult or fad such as vegetarianism or crash dieting.'[14]

Adolescence is a period of rapid physical growth and change. Enormous growth spurts are reflected by corresponding surges in appetite. Many levels of nutrients required by the growing teenager are considerably higher in proportion to body size and weight than they will be in adult years. Adolescence is also a period of emotional and psychological change, when the independent character of the individual is established. There is a tendency to reject convention and to exert independence by making individual decisions. Food choice is one of the first targets, teenagers often choosing unconventional meals and odd combinations of food. More meals are now eaten outside the home and unbalanced meals may be chosen from the vast array of take-away food outlets. Meals are frequently missed, particularly breakfast, which can lead to a heavy reliance on snack items. Many convenience snack items tend to be high in 'empty' calories – that is, they contain plenty of calories but little in the way of essential nutrients because of their high fat and sugar contents. However, it is not sensible to ban such items totally from the diet as many teenagers would not be able to meet their energy requirements without them. They should not take the place of more nutrient-dense foods, but should be used as a 'top-up' to an already balanced diet. The teenage years see the start of alcohol consumption which is also of great concern.

Energy. Many teenagers go through a phase of eating much more than adults, especially around the time of their peak height velocity (growth spurt). Energy needs will also vary with the amount of physical activity undertaken. Inactive teenagers may become obese even though their energy intake is below recommendations, whereas extremely active young people will have greater needs than those recommended. Energy needs should be adjusted to balance energy expenditure.

Protein. Protein supplies a constant 12–14 per cent of total energy intake throughout childhood and adolescence. The peak in protein intake coincides with the peak in energy intake. So, although protein intake is important, the quantity of food necessary to meet the energy needs of the individual will come with more than enough protein.

There is in fact very little evidence of insufficient protein intakes. Energy intakes may fall below needs in those limiting their food intake (usually to reduce bodyweight). However, when energy is limited, dietary protein is used to meet the energy needs and is therefore not available for synthesis of new tissue. The result is a fall-off in growth rate even though the protein intake appears adequate.

Minerals. The minerals most likely to be inadequately supplied in the teenage diet are calcium, iron and zinc. There is an increased need for all these minerals during growth spurts – calcium because of the increase in skeletal mass, iron because of the expansion of muscle mass and blood volume, and zinc because of the generation of both skeletal and muscle tissue.

Calcium. Accretion of calcium in the skeleton can be as much as 100 g per year at peak height velocity (growth spurt).[5] Only around 20 per cent of dietary calcium is absorbed so that 500 g is needed in the yearly diet – that is 1370 mg/day. Unless dairy products are consumed regularly, it is very difficult to provide sufficient calcium in the diet. It is also important to remember that calcium from vegetables is poorly absorbed by the body. Osteoporosis (brittle bones) is an example of the origins of an adult disease beginning in childhood. The severity of bone loss occurring in women after the menopause is partly determined by the skeletal development in the teenage years. Bone density is increased when girls have a diet adequate in calcium and take regular exercise. The table below lists calcium-rich foods and how much calcium can be derived from what quantities of them. It is followed by some practical suggestions of how to increase calcium intake.

Calcium-rich Foods

	Dietary Source	Calcium Content mg
Dairy Produce	1 pint whole milk	690
	1 pint semi-skimmed milk	720
	1 pint skimmed milk	750
	1 oz cheese (Cheddar)	220
	5 oz pot yoghurt	255

Calcium-rich Foods

	Dietary Source	Calcium Content mg
Cereals	2 slices white bread	60
	2 slices wholemeal bread	14
Fish	2 oz sardines (including bones)	220
Vegetables and Pulses	4 oz cabbage	57
	4 oz broccoli	76
	1 oz watercress	45
	4 oz baked beans	60
Nuts	2 oz peanuts	34
Fruit	2 oz dried apricots	50
	4 oz oranges	50
Ice-cream	2 oz dairy ice-cream	78

How to increase calcium intake:

1. Milk and cereal taken together increase the absorption of calcium from the cereal.
2. An adequate supply of vitamin D is essential for calcium absorption – obtained from the action of sunlight on the skin, oily fish, margarine, butter and eggs.
3. Five or six cups of hard tap water can supply up to 200 mg calcium per day.
4. White bread has a higher calcium content than wholemeal because calcium is added by law to all flours except wholemeal.
5. Smoking, alcohol drinking and stress all increase the requirement for calcium.
6. High protein intake leads to increased loss of calcium via the urine.
7. A high calcium intake is not harmful for the vast majority because any excess is not absorbed into the bloodstream.

Iron. Iron deficiency is quite common in adolescent girls who are menstruating, still growing and often restricting their food intake. It may sometimes occur in boys too, during periods of rapid growth and irregular or inadequate diet. Iron deficiency anaemia is by far the most common form of anaemia encountered in general practice. Iron status can be improved by including good sources of iron in the diet. Iron is better absorbed from some foods than others and, in addition, some dietary constituents may impair or facilitate absorption. Here is a list of iron-rich foods and ways of increasing iron intake.

Iron-rich Foods

	Dietary Source	*Iron content (mg)*
Meat	4 oz liver	12.0
	2 oz kidney	7.2
	2 oz black pudding	12.0
	6 oz grilled steak	6.3
	2 oz corned beef	1.7
Fish	2 oz sardines	2.8
	2 oz cockles	15.6
	2 oz mussels	4.6
Eggs	1 size 3 egg	1.2
Cereals	2 slices white bread	1.5
	2 slices wholemeal bread	1.0
	1 oz All Bran	3.6
	1 oz muesli	1.4
	1 oz Weetabix	2.3
Vegetables	6 oz potatoes – baked	1.4
	4 oz cabbage	0.6
	1 oz watercress	0.5
Fruit	2 oz dried apricots	2.5
Nuts	2 oz almonds	2.5
	2 oz peanuts	1.2

How to increase iron intake:

1. Haem iron (in meat and offal) is better absorbed than non-haem iron (in cereals, fruit, nuts and vegetables).
2. Absorption of non-haem iron can be improved by eating vitamin C-rich foods at the same meal, e.g., citrus fruit, green leafy vegetables.

3. Spinach is very rich in iron but the iron is not easily absorbed.
4. For most people, iron supplements are not harmful. If there is no shortage, iron will not be absorbed, but regular over dosing can lead to poisoning.

Zinc. Zinc is an essential mineral for growth and sexual development. Retention is markedly increased during the growth spurt, but adolescents still have high requirements for this mineral. These can be met with extra meat, milk and fish.

A sensible diet for teenagers. A healthy diet should be based on as wide a variety of foods as possible, with emphasis on nutrient-dense foods rather than those which provide energy but relatively few essential nutrients. The table below shows how food can be chosen from the different food groups (p. 177) to provide the necessary nutrients. Total quantities of food will need to be altered to allow for the wide variation in appetite and energy requirement between teenagers of different age and sex. Tact, patience and understanding are required in large measures by both parents and teachers if teenagers are to be steered towards a pattern of sensible healthy eating and away from extreme diets with potentially harmful consequences.

Suggested Daily Eating Plan for Teenagers

Food Group	Daily Servings
Group One	4 or more to satisfy appetite.
Group Two	4 or more.
Group Three	2–3
Group Four	4 or more.
Group Five	In addition to basic foods, not as substitutes. Take care if there is a tendency to put excess weight on.
Group Six	In small amounts.

Snacking. Adolescents are great snackers. For some, snacks may provide the majority of their energy needs for the day. Therefore, it is essential that these snacks provide basic nutrients and energy.

Many convenience snack foods are high in fat, sugar and/or salt and fail to provide adequate amounts of protein, vitamins, minerals and dietary fibre. Tasty and convenient snacks which are also nutritious are: wholemeal cracker biscuits, low fat cheese, wholemeal bread or rolls, pizza, wholemeal cereals, dried fruit and nuts, fresh fruit, semi-skimmed milk, low fat yoghurt, wholemeal fruit buns, peanut butter on bread or crackers. Because of the high energy requirement of some adolescents, some 'empty calorie' snack foods can be consumed, as top-ups to the balanced diet. However, snacking on such foods should not become a habit, as it will be necessary to eliminate these foods when growth ceases and the overall energy requirement drops.

Fast foods. Adolescents find fast foods very attractive and they often meet at their local fast-food outlet. Many, but not all, take-aways are high in fat, sugar and salt, and a heavy reliance on such foods may lead to nutritional inadequacies. Careful selection of take-aways can provide a well-balanced meal: hamburgers with plenty of salad; vegetarian wholemeal pizza; jacket potato instead of chips or french fries; a glass of milk rather than a thick sweet milkshake; fruit juice rather than sugary, fizzy drinks.

Dietary supplements. A study in 1988 indicated that non-verbal intelligence might be increased by multi-vitamin and mineral supplementation.[6] While these findings were of interest and worth further investigation, the study received widespread scientific criticism. Until further evidence proves the contrary, there would seem no merit in supplementing the diet of teenagers provided they are consuming a varied range of foods, and unless there is a specific medical need for an additional vitamin or mineral supplement.

Vegetarianism. Adolescents may adopt a vegetarian, vegan or macrobiotic style of eating for religious, moral, health or ecological reasons. Four classes of vegetarianism are recognized: semi-vegetarians who eat no red meat; lacto-ovo vegetarians who eat no meat or fish but do eat dairy products and eggs; lacto-vegetarians who eat dairy products but no eggs, meat or fish; total vegetarians or vegans who eat nothing of animal origin. The extent of nutritional risk from these diets will depend on the range of foods that is excluded. When planning a vegetarian diet for a teenager, the higher level of nutrient and energy requirements compared to those of adults must be taken into account. Teenagers following a vegan diet will need to take special care of their vitamin B_{12} intake by consuming foods that naturally contain the vitamin (edible seaweeds and tempeh) or fortified foods (most yeast extracts, some soya milks, cereals and margarines and textured vegetable protein) or vitamin supplements. Because of the high demand for calcium in adolescence and because the calcium from plant sources is relatively poorly absorbed, calcium supplements may also be required. Protein intake should not be inadequate in the vegan diet provided cereal, pulse, and green vegetable sources are combined to ensure the right mix of amino acids at each meal. However, because of the bulky nature of such diets, some teenagers may find it difficult to consume enough food to supply the relatively high energy needs. It is important to monitor the growth of such children.

Weight control. Most obese adults become obese for the first time during their adolescent years. Obesity affects approximately 10 per cent of all male and female adolescents, and as in adults, should be seen as an imbalance between energy intake and energy expenditure. Evidence from Australia and the United States indicates that the decrease in physical activity may be an important factor in adolescent obesity.[7] This decline in activity is also apparent in the UK. Height gain is an important factor in adolescent weight control. Adolescents gain approximately 5 lb of bone and muscle for every inch of growth. If weight is maintained while growth increases, body fat percentage will fall, i.e. they will 'grow out' of their fatness. Severe energy restriction is not advisable for growing adolescents as a drastic weight loss can jeopardize health and the attainment of full growth. Restricting food intake below requirements will also lead to the development of iron-deficiency anaemia and other nutrition-related conditions. Foods such as bread, potatoes, lean meats, fish, fruit and vegetables should not be restricted. The high-energy foods which provide much less in the way of nutrients such as fried foods, pastries, sweets, chocolates and sugary, fizzy drinks should be avoided. In serious cases of overweight, or when weight stabilization is not being achieved during periods of rapid growth, advice should be sought from a doctor or dietician (or both).

Anorexia nervosa and bulimia nervosa

Adolescent females sometimes modify their diet because they are not as thin as they, or their peers, think they should be. To achieve this they may also fast and binge alternately. With a smaller energy intake they are less likely to reach their requirements for iron and other essential nutrients. In a small minority this social dieting leads to anorexia nervosa. This is a psychological illness, affecting primarily adolescent girls and young women, usually middle class and of above average intelligence. The problem is believed to lie both in a fear of normal adolescent bodyweight, and in difficulties in accepting that the biological changes accompanying adult sexuality are important. Treatment of anorexia nervosa is best handled by a specialist team including a psychiatrist and a dietician. It is important to recognize the condition early, as the longer the duration, the worse the prognosis. A young woman with a body mass index of less than 18 (weight (kg)/height (m)^2) should be warned, with her parents, that her thinness is unhealthy, and she should be referred for treatment if she cannot increase it. By contrast, adolescent boys are more likely to worry that they are not growing tall enough, or not developing enough muscles.

Symptoms of anorexia nervosa:

1. Continuing weight loss.
2. Increasingly skeletal appearance – protrusion of shoulder blades, backbone, bones on hips and buttocks. Sitting for any length of time on a hard surface becomes uncomfortable.
3. Regular self-weighing.
4. Disturbed body-image – complaining of feeling 'fat' even when emaciated.
5. Hyperactivity and obsession with exercise.
6. Restless sleep and early waking. (Animals who are hungry prowl restlessly in search of food rather than sleeping.)
7. Cessation of periods (amenorrhoea).
8. Blueish-mauve colouring at extremities, which could also be cold to the touch (acrocyanosis).
9. Abuse of laxatives and diuretics.
10. Loner behaviour and insistence that, despite displaying many of the above symptoms, all is well.

There may also be other symptoms such as rough skin, constipation, oedema, dizziness and weakness etc., due simply to a dietary deficiency.

Bulimia nervosa is another psychological condition. It causes powerful urges to overeat, but overweight is avoided by vomiting, purgatives and periods of starvation. Bulimics are often shy, hardworking women who keep their problem to themselves. The binge foods are usually sweet and starchy and huge amounts can be eaten at one time. Many young women suffering from bulimia are former anorexia nervosa sufferers. As with anorexia nervosa, bulimia nervosa has nutritional repercussions but, although the treatment of this disorder has a dietary component, the main approach is one of psychotherapy.

Warning signs of bulimia nervosa:

1. General obsession with food.
2. Unusually frequent visits to the bathroom or toilet after or between meals to 'wash my hair' or 'take a quick shower'.
3. Traces of vomit in the toilet or bathroom.
4. Poor condition of sufferer's teeth – where the acidic action of vomiting erodes tooth enamel and decay follows.
5. Disappearance of food from cupboard and refrigerator.
6. Fluctuations of weight over short periods of time.
7. Sufferer often short of money, having spent it on clandestine food.
8. Frequent self-weighing.
9. Unexplained cake, biscuit, and sweet wrappings around the house – under pillows, mattress and chairs.
10. Disinterest in social activities, preferring to stay at home.
11. Staying up alone at night, often for further binge/purge.
12. Habit developing of short, impromptu walks – in the direction of food shops.

(Reference: *Too Thin To Win* – an information booklet on eating disorders, produced under the auspices of the International Athletic Foundation, 1989. Available from IAAF, 3 Hans Crescent, London SW1.)

Sports nutrition for children

Strenuous physical activity, training and athletic competition do not appear significantly to alter the requirement for any specific nutrient except calories and water. There is no increase in the requirement for protein, vitamins and minerals that cannot be met best through a food intake that satisfies the energy needs of the active young athlete.

Energy. The most prevalent nutrition-related problem among young athletes is meeting their energy needs.[8] The amount of energy required will depend on age, growth status, and type, duration and intensity of exercise. Very athletic 7–10-year-olds may need 3000–4000 kcals per day, while very athletic adolescents may need as much as 5000 kcals. This compares with a Recommended Daily Amount (RDA) of 1900–2000 kcals for ordinary 7–10-year-olds and 2150–2880 kcals for ordinary adolescents.[1] For active children the proportion of energy coming from the various components of the diet should be: 55 per cent carbohydrate, 15 per cent protein and 30 per cent fat.

Carbohydrate and fat. The storage form of carbohydrate in the body is glycogen. It is stored in the muscles and liver and is a readily available source of energy for the body. Only glycogen stored in the muscles that are actually exercising can be used to supply energy to those muscles. Once that glycogen store is depleted, the muscles will become fatigued and performance will fall off. Liver glycogen is used mainly to maintain the blood glucose levels needed to supply the vital organs such as the nervous system.

The body uses both carbohydrate (glycogen) and fat (triglycerides) as fuel, and their relative contributions depend on the intensity and duration of exercise, and the state of physical training. At low exercise intensities, such as jogging, a proportion of energy is provided by carbohydrate and fat together. As exercise intensity increases, such as switching to running, the contribution of energy production from carbohydrate rises and that from fat falls. When there is a rapid demand for energy, as in sprinting, carbohydrate provides most if not all of the energy.

The amount of fat stored in the body is so vast that lack of fat is virtually never a cause of fatigue. Stored carbohydrate is so meagre that lack of muscle glycogen and liver glycogen are frequently limiting factors in athletic events that require endurance. Indeed, whatever the sport undertaken, if carbohydrate is not replaced after each event, the athlete will eventually suffer from residual fatigue and performance will fall off. Eating foods high in carbohydrate as soon as possible after exercise is vital to prevent glycogen depletion. Conversion of food to muscle glycogen is most efficient during the first hour after exercise – unfortunately, a time when most athletes feel least like eating. Foods or drinks with high carbohydrate content should therefore be consumed as soon as it is feasible. Use the tables below to work out how best to get the carbohydrates needed after exercise.

Grams Carbohydrate to be Supplied on Various Energy Intakes

Total Energy	Percentage Total Energy from Carbohydrate			
	45% grams	50% grams	55% grams	60% grams
2000 kcals	225	250	275	300
3000 kcals	335	375	410	450
4000 kcals	450	500	550	600
5000 kcals	560	625	685	750

Quantities of Food Containing Approximately 10 Grams Carbohydrate

	Food	Portion containing 10 g sugar or starch
Sugar	White or brown	2 level tsp
	Boiled sweets	$\frac{1}{3}$ oz
	Jam, honey, marmalade	1 tsp
	Toffees	$\frac{1}{2}$ oz
	Chocolate	$\frac{2}{3}$ oz
Cereals	Flour	1 level tbsp
	Unsweetened breakfast cereals	3 heaped tbsp
	Boiled rice	1 tbsp
	Boiled pasta	2 tbsp
	Bread (any kind)	$\frac{1}{2}$ large slice
	Crispbread	$\frac{1}{2}$ oz
	Cream crackers	2 biscuits
	Sweet biscuits	2 'plain' type
	Shortcrust pastry	$\frac{2}{3}$ oz
	Scones	$\frac{2}{3}$ oz
Fruit	Currants, dates, sultanas, raisins	$\frac{1}{2}$ oz
	Peeled bananas	$\frac{1}{2}$ large one

	Food	Portion containing 10 g sugar or starch
	Grapes, tinned fruit	2 oz
	Raspberries, strawberries	6 oz
	Most other fruit	e.g. 1 medium apple
Vegetables	Lentils and dried pulses	$\frac{2}{3}$ oz
	Chips	4 large ones
	Boiled potatoes	2 oz
	Baked beans, sweetcorn	2 oz
	Boiled parsnips	$2\frac{1}{2}$ oz
	Boiled beetroot	1 medium one
	Boiled peas, broad beans	4 tbsp
	Boiled carrots	*Large* portion

Most other vegetables are virtually carbohydrate-free.

Dairy foods	Milk	1 glass
	Low fat, unsweetened yoghurt	1 individual pot
	Cottage Cheese	8 oz

Other cheeses, butter and cream are virtually carbohydrate-free.

Meat, fish, eggs	Sausages	$2\frac{1}{2}$ oz

Fresh meat, fish (except some shellfish) and eggs are carbohydrate-free.

Beverages	Fruit juice, unsweetened	4 fl oz

Others	Ice cream	1 small brick
	Peanuts, shelled	4 oz

Fats and oils are carbohydrate-free.

Made-up and manufactured products are very variable in content. Booklets containing information about brand products are available from supermarkets.

(Adapted from *The Everyman Companion to Food and Nutrition*, Sheila Bingham, 1987. Published by J. M. Dent & Sons Ltd.)

Protein. Physical training, not protein, increases muscle mass. Yet high protein diets remain popular among many athletes. Such athletes reason that there must be a need for an increased protein intake to synthesize the additional muscle protein. However, a number of studies have shown that a daily protein intake of approximately 1 g/kg b.wt. (i.e., what the average adult eats) is sufficient in young men undergoing athletic training. Although the protein requirement for adolescents is slightly higher than that for young men, a daily intake of 1–1.5 g/kg in relation to bodyweight (b.wt.) of high quality animal protein should be sufficient to meet the needs of young adolescents (male and female) in training.[9]

The balanced, mixed Western diet supplies roughly 15 per cent of total energy as protein. If the extra energy requirement of exercise is met by such a diet, extra protein will also be supplied in the diet and the young athlete will be getting at least 2 g/kg b.wt. protein a day. A mixture of protein should be included in the diet. Animal protein is often accompanied by large amounts of fat which can push out the much-needed carbohydrate. The diet must contain vegetable sources of protein as well. Protein supplements should not be necessary. The table below lists animal and vegetable protein sources.

Approximate Protein Content of some Average Portions of Food

Type of Food	Grams Protein	Average Portion
Fish	18	100 g steamed cod
Meat, poultry	13	50 g lean roast beef
Cheese	12	50 g cheddar
Milk	10	Half a pint
Egg	7	1 grade three
Nuts	14	50 g peanuts
Pulses	8	150 g can baked beans
Cereals	8	3 thin slices bread
Vegetables	2	Av. portion (150 g) potatoes
Fruit	$\frac{1}{2}$	1 medium apple

Iron. The adequacy of iron stores in children who are training has received much attention – understandably, as apart from during pregnancy and breast-feeding, the dietary requirement for iron is greatest between the ages of 12 and 16 years. Overt iron deficiency results in anaemia, but lesser levels of iron depletion may affect cognitive, gastrointestinal and immunological function. Moreover, there is evidence that non-anaemic iron deficiency may impair athletic performance.[10]

Iron deficiency is known to affect at least 10–20 per cent of women of fertile age in Western countries. The iron intakes of many adolescent girls are very low, putting them at high risk of iron deficiency, particularly if they have heavy menstrual losses.[11] Almost half of female adolescent endurance athletes can be expected to have low iron stores[10] and female adolescent dancers show a similar picture.[12] Since iron deficiency – iron depletion and anaemia – are common in adolescent female athletes, periodic evaluation of iron status should be carried out. If iron supplements are used, they should not exceed the RDA unless there is a strong indication for additional iron. As more adolescents eat less red meat and either become vegetarians or consume more fish and poultry (which contain less iron than red meat), attention must be paid to the iron content of the diet (see the table on p. 191).

Fluid. Young athletes who are pre-pubescent or in the early stages of puberty can have fluid balance and thermoregulation problems which are often not appreciated by their coaches or people supervising them. When exercising in heat, these athletes cannot keep their body temperature down as well as adults, because the sweat glands of their skin are not yet fully developed. They are also less able to adapt to periods of prolonged sweating or to acclimatize to the heat as effectively as adults. On the other hand, heat is quickly lost in colder environments, particularly in water. To make matters worse, it has been found that younger athletes are able to develop a sense of well-being more rapidly than older athletes when exercising in the heat. This psychological adjustment to the warm environment is not met by a complete physiological adjustment, and this increases the risk of heat-induced problems. Children, like adults, do not voluntarily replenish all fluid losses during exercise.

Enough fluid should be consumed to replace fluids lost in perspiration and to prevent dehydration. This applies to all active children, from very young girls in ballet classes to adolescent boys training and playing football regularly. To prevent dehydration, coaches and parents should encourage liberal fluid intake, before, during and after vigorous exercise. Depending on the duration and intensity of the exercise, between 200 ml and 500 ml of water should be drunk between twenty and forty minutes before, and small amounts of fluid taken little and often during exercise, when the particular sport allows. Following exercise the re-hydration process should be started straight away. The most important consideration throughout is fluid intake, so plain water is the first choice, or alternatively dilute fruit juice if this is preferred. Commercial drinks,

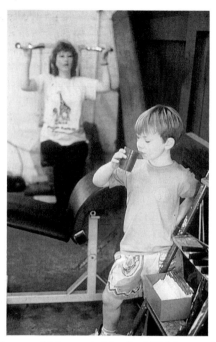

Frequent drinks are vital for the child doing exercise.

if used with care, can assist in replacing fluid loss and at the same time can provide additional carbohydrate to supplement the body's energy reserves. However, if used incorrectly they may cause nausea and stomach discomfort, and can affect performance. Salt tablets are to be avoided at all costs. It should also go without saying that fluid restriction should *not* be used to control bodyweight.

Practical applications. Nutritional intake varies considerably in quantity and quality among young athletes. In general, athletes do not select diets that promote best performance or health. An inadequate or incorrect diet will undercut much of the hard effort of training.

The diet of physically active children should still be based around the Basic Food Groups (see p. 177). A suggested plan for one day is:

Four servings from Group One.
Four servings from Group Two.
Two servings from Group Three.
Two servings from Group Four.

Quantities will be determined by the child's age and energy needs. Some adolescents will need more servings from Groups Three and Four to ensure adequate intakes of iron and calcium, but the bulk of the diet should come from Groups One and Two to ensure sufficient intake of carbohydrate. This may still be inadequate for young athletes (children and adolescents) with particularly high energy requirements. So for these, second helpings and 'preference' foods should be added to the basic diet to satisfy energy needs and maintain desired bodyweight. Preference foods will probably include sweets, chocolate, cakes, biscuits, honey and jams and 'straight' sugar. These should be seen as 'top-ups' to the diet and should not replace the more nutrient-dense foods. A good maxim for an active child is 'eat what you need, *then* what you want'.

Weight control. Some athletes request (though do not necessarily require) dietary advice to enable them to lose weight. The most effective way to lose weight is to combine a period of controlled energy intake and a sensible programme of endurance activity into the normal training programme. The aim of all such dietary regimes is to restrict the food intake so that the body's stores of fat are used to make up the energy deficit. It is very important to keep up the carbohydrate content of the diet and to make up the diet with nutrient-dense foods which will continue to provide the essential nutrients. Fatty foods should be avoided as these are particularly high in calories. Here are suggestions for ways of avoiding fat.

How to cut back fat intake:

1. Use a low fat spread rather than butter or margarine, especially as the bread intake should not be cut back.
2. Use semi-skimmed milk rather than whole milk.
3. Use low fat cheeses or cottage cheese rather than full fat cheeses.
4. Eat fish or chicken but avoid the chicken skin as this is fatty.
5. Remove fat from red meat or buy lean cuts when possible.
6. Grill, steam of microwave food rather than frying, and drain off any fat that appears during cooking.
7. Use natural yoghurt, lemon juice and herbs instead of mayonnaise or creamy sauces.
8. Choose dishes which combine meat with pasta, beans or

vegetables. This reduces the fat and increases the carbohydrate of the dish.

9. Use low fat alternatives when available, e.g., when choosing sausages, hamburgers.
10. Keep the proportion of starchy carbohydrates up, e.g., breads, cereals, vegetables, pulses and fruit.

The practice of starving to achieve a rapid weight loss in the days before a weight-class sport competition is well known. Other methods include pushing up the amount of exercise, restricting specific foods, cutting back fluid intake, or increasing fluid loss by wearing sweat suits, training in hot environments and using diuretics. Potential risks exist for young athletes involved in these practices. Starvation leads to loss of lean body mass. Because the thermoregulatory mechanism in young athletes is not as effective as in adults, they are potentially at greater risk from heat-related problems. There may be serious long-term effects if these practices are repeated often.

Weight control in the young female athlete. The young female athlete faces difficult problems and choices in trying simultaneously to juggle growth, strength, weight and optimal body fat. The result is often a conscious act to reduce food intake. The post-pubertal female gains fat naturally, while her sport may demand unnatural thinness. The fat that is being laid down may be seen as undesirable by the individual and her coach. Other young females believe that weight loss will enhance performance. This tends to happen in a girl who starts out a little overweight. As she wins and improves she links this to her weight loss and so strives to bring her weight down even further.

At first, food intake is reduced and there is usually a heavy reliance on low energy-dense foods which are bulky, e.g., salads, vegetables and fruit. A profound and deliberate restriction of food may ultimately lead to an actual aversion to food itself and the manifestations of anorexia nervosa. At this stage diet pills, laxatives, diuretics, self-induced vomiting and a cycle of bingeing and starving may be used to achieve greater weight losses. The facts about these methods are stark:

1. They impair performance, not improve it, by inducing dehydration and malnutrition.

2. They have serious short- and long-term consequences, e.g., osteoporosis, stress fractures, loss of dental enamel, oligomenorrhoea and amenorrhoea (partial and complete loss of menstruation), cardiac arrhythmias, gastrointestinal problems, oesophageal tears and crucial electrolyte and fluid imbalances.
3. They have serious psychological consequences, e.g., mood swings, depression, guilt, shame, etc.
4. They do not cause effective weight loss as fluid and muscle or lean body mass are lost as well.

See the list of symptoms of anorexia nervosa on p. 195.

Eating for competition. The basic principles for eating to maximize exercise performance apply equally to children, adolescents and adults. They apply equally to males and females and across the board for all sports.[13]

Many adolescents take nutritional supplements in the hope that these will improve their ability to compete in sports. No supplement will improve athletic performance unless it replaces a nutrient that is not available in the athlete's diet or is not present in sufficient amounts to meet requirements. For example, vitamin supplements have not been shown to enhance performance, reduce injury rates or promote recovery from injury.

Many young athletes do not appreciate the importance of replenishing glycogen stores after each training session and event. Consequently they have glycogen stores which are inadequate to support an all-out effort for their entire event, particularly in an endurance sport. Carbohydrate loading is practised by some endurance athletes, but it is not recommended for adolescents. It is a way of increasing the store of glycogen in the muscles. For the first three days of the week preceding a marathon the athlete will eat a low carbohydrate diet and will exercise very hard. For the rest of the week to the race the athlete will switch to a high carbohydrate diet and will taper exercise right down. There are disadvantages in this technique, and it has not been shown to be more effective than simply reducing the work load and eating more carbohydrates. For an endurance event, training should be reduced significantly for the three days before the event and regular meals should be eaten with extra carbohydrate snacks in-between.

A Typical High-carbohydrate Day

Breakfast	Muesli or other wholegrain cereal, dried fruit and semi-skimmed milk. Wholemeal toast, rolls, muffins with jam, marmalade, honey or peanut butter. Fresh fruit juice. Tea and coffee or milk.
Mid-morning	Wholegrain cereal and fruit bar; fruit (fresh or dried). Tea, coffee, milk or fruit juice.
Lunch	Wholemeal sandwiches (filling based around meat, fish, cheese, eggs, peanut butter or bananas) and salad *or* baked beans, pizza or bean and pasta dish and salad. Fresh or dried fruit, yoghurt *or* 'simple' cake or biscuit (e.g., flapjack, gingerbread, fruit cake or digestive biscuits). Fruit juice, tea, coffee, milk or water.
Mid-afternoon	As mid-morning.
Evening meal	Plenty of vegetables including beans and peas. Potatoes, pasta or rice. Meat, fish, poultry, cheese, eggs, nuts. Pudding as at lunch or fruit crumble or pie or milk pudding.
Bedtime (if hungry)	Milky drink. Sandwich with low fat filling *or* a bowl of breakfast cereal and milk.

The night before a competition. A high carbohydrate meal the night before competition provides the last opportunity to push up the glycogen content of the muscles as the pre-competition meal next morning is too close to the event to be effective in doing this. (For competitions that take place in the late afternoon or evening, a high carbohydrate meal can be eaten in the morning.) There is no evidence that simple sugars are less effective than starches in maximizing muscle glycogen stores. Suggested foods for this meal include:

Pasta and tomato sauce.

Bread roll.

Milk to drink or fruit juice. (Many athletes prefer to avoid gassy drinks at this stage for obvious reasons.)

Ice-cream, fruit pie or crumble and custard or simple cake such as fruit cake, gingerbread or flapjacks.

Pre-competition meal. This meal should be planned well in advance and not left to the last moment. Its function is to maximize the liver (not muscle) glycogen and to stop the competitor feeling hungry. The timing of the meal is more important than the content. It should not be eaten less than two to three hours before the event. Some individuals find that they cannot tolerate food less than five hours before. Any preferred food can be eaten as long as there is no discomfort and the stomach is empty before the start. This rules out high fat foods as they take the longest to leave the stomach. Light, carbohydrate foods appear to be the best choice. Often an individual has a preference for a food that he or she believes helps performance. Provided it fits into the above guidelines, this should be permitted. Some athletes benefit from taking a commercial liquid drink, though others suffer from cramps and diarrhoea after them. This highlights the importance of experimenting with different foods and preparations in training sessions and not trying things out for the first time at important events. A simple carbohydrate meal could include cereal and milk, toast and jam, honey or peanut butter and plenty of fluid. Although this sounds like a breakfast, it makes an excellent pre-competition meal at any time of the day.

Food and drink during competition. Young athletes will always benefit from keeping adequately hydrated. Competitive adolescent runners and swimmers can lose approximately 1.5 litres of fluid during an intense one-hour workout.[13] Although athletes exercising in warm humid conditions can see their sweat and appreciate the fluid loss, those exercising in water may not be able to recognize that this loss is happening. Athletes should drink before they feel thirsty, as dehydration is already underway if feelings of thirst are experienced. Cold water is the first choice and should be drunk before the event and at regular intervals throughout.

It is not necessary for most adolescents to eat during events that last less than two hours, but they can benefit from having an intake of carbohydrate during events that last longer. The choice is mostly one of personal preference and what an individual can tolerate, but commercial sports drinks are favoured by many athletes. It is important to choose a drink that is isotonic (has a concentration similar to that of body fluid) and contains carbohydrate polymers (maltodextrin). Such a drink will increase both carbohydrate and fluid intake. The label on the product will supply the information needed to make a choice of the most suitable drink. Dietary changes, such as drinking a new sports drink, should always be tested in training first and never in competition.

After competition. Recovery from exercise depends on the replenishment of glycogen stores. It makes no difference whether this is done by consuming starchy or simple carbohydrates, so again the 'preference' foods (see p. 203) should be chosen as they will be tolerated sooner than others. In events such as gymnastics, track and field events, wrestling, boxing and swimming, athletes may have to compete in several events in one day. It is very important for them to drink immediately after they finish each event and to eat as soon as they can. The quantities and nature of the food will be dictated by the time interval between each event:

Two or more hours	Sandwiches, milk and fruit.
One to two hours	Liquid meals of eggs, milk, bananas, yoghurt etc.
Less than one hour	Juice, soft drinks, confectionery and commercial preparations.

Competing away from home. It is advisable to check out the eating arrangements in advance. Contingency plans can then be made to provide the athlete with the types of food he or she is used to eating before, during and after an event if they are not going to be available. If travelling abroad, familiar packeted or canned food such as a favourite breakfast cereal can be taken from the home country. This is especially important when the event is taking place in a country with very different eating habits and foods from home.

Useful Addresses

ANOREXIC AID
The Priory Centre,
11 Priory Road, High Wycombe,
Buckinghamshire, HP13 6SL.

ANOREXIC FAMILY AID
Sackville Place,
44 Magdalen Street,
Norwich, Norfolk, NR3 1JE.

BRITISH DIETETIC ASSOCIATION
7th Floor, Elizabeth House,
22 Suffolk Street, Queensway,
Birmingham B1 1LS.

HYPERACTIVE CHILDREN'S
SUPPORT GROUP
71 Whyke Lane,
Chichester,
West Sussex, PO19 2LI.

NATIONAL COACHING
FOUNDATION INFORMATION
SERVICE
4 College Close,
Beckett Park,
Leeds LS6 3QH.

NATIONAL SOCIETY FOR
RESEARCH INTO ALLERGY
PO Box 45,
Hinckley,
Leicestershire, LE10 1JY.

SPORTS NUTRITION FOUNDATION
London Sports Medicine
Institute,
c/o Medical College of St.
Bartholomew's Hospital,
Charterhouse Square,
London EC1M 6BQ.
(Provides advice, comment and
literature on sports nutrition for
anyone involved in competitive
and recreational sport at all
levels.)

SPORTS NUTRITION SERVICE
Department of Physical
Education and Sports Science,
Loughborough University,
Loughborough,
Leicestershire, LE11 3TU.
(Provides a dietary analysis
service for all national and
County level athletes.)

VEGAN SOCIETY
7 Battle Road,
St. Leonards-on-Sea,
East Sussex, TN37 7AA.

VEGETARIAN SOCIETY
Parkdale, Dunham Road,
Altrincham,
Cheshire, WA14 4QG.

12 Conclusions

The current writers make no secret of favouring sport and exercise for children. We believe that sport and exercise can contribute essential benefits, including healthy growth of the bones and soft tissues, and good postural muscle tone. If the child learns to enjoy exercise from an early age, healthy exercise habits are established which can form the basis of physical well-being and health-related fitness throughout adult life and well into old age. Sport and exercise improve a child's co-ordination and physical skills. They carry additional, less quantifiable benefits, such as improving the child's confidence and self-esteem, and providing a context in which the child can meet other children, as well as adults, and learn to socialize, form friendships, and cope with rivalries. If the sport involves travel to other towns, places or countries, it broadens the child's horizons.

Healthy growth also depends on an appropriate diet, so it is important to establish healthy eating patterns in childhood, even though the details of what constitutes a healthy diet will change as the child gets older.

Very young children may take physical exercise simply through playing active games. Teenagers might take their exercise in the form of disco dancing. All children should be encouraged to be active every day, especially in preference to excessive television viewing. Through play or dance, exercise can form a natural part of the child's recreational activities. If sport and exercise form part of the family's routine, the child's physical activities take on a more organized aspect. Some children may need encouraging and per-suading to be active, especially if they find sports difficult, or if they feel they are not particularly talented for any form of exercise. As the parent or responsible adult you should create opportunities for sports and exercise for the child that are as widely varied as possible. The child should also have opportunities for other interests appropriate for the age-group. Activities such as reading, listening to music, bird-watching, making models, joining the Cubs, Brownies, Boys' Brigade, Scouts or Girl Guides, or more esoteric pastimes like bell-ringing, can be encouraged alongside sports, rather than as alternatives. A wide choice prevents boredom, and gives the child a chance of finding at least some activities enjoyable. Encouragement and persuasion should never lead you to force the child to do activities he or she dislikes.

Specialization is an essential factor if the child is aiming at high-level competition or a professional career. We believe that early specialization and over-specialization should be discouraged. Apart from the risk of disappointment and 'burn-out' should the child fail to achieve success, there are serious risks of injury and distorted body development if the child is encouraged or allowed to do one sport to the exclusion of all others. Every sport done at competitive level requires background fitness training, and an important part of training is protective exercise to counterbalance the particular sport's possible harmful stresses. Protective and postural exercises are the only type of physical training which could and should remain

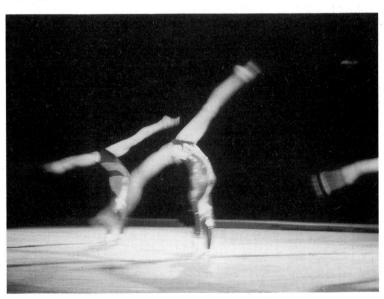

Female gymnasts need to be strong, supple and lightweight.

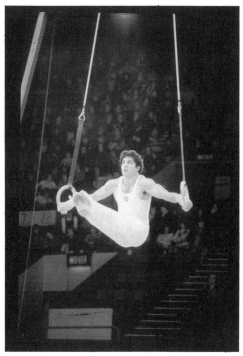

Male gymnasts have to be strong.

constant from earliest childhood to old age.

The skills of any sport are best learned at a young age, but the skills have to be adapted as the child grows, and the child has to adjust to changes of technique. This is why it is difficult to predict whether the child who has been successful in junior competitions will necessarily be a winner at senior level, and why, equally, success can come to competitors who are late starters in a sport. Female gymnastics is one of the very few sports restricted at its top level to young competitors. As it involves very long hours of training and total commitment, it is not enough for the child to be keen and reasonably talented: you have to be certain that the child is totally suited to the sport before allowing her to become engrossed in it beyond the recreational level. Success can also come to young competitors in other sports. Where sports like tennis offer high earning levels to successful professionals, the responsible adult (parent, manager or coach) has to assess and resist the pressures and dangers, because the successful teenager can all too easily be lured or forced into playing matches when ill, injured or over-fatigued, with possible long-term harm.

In most sports, competitors do not normally reach the top before the late teens or early twenties, when they have virtually reached physical maturity. In some sports, such as running, tennis, rowing, karate, cricket and golf, competitors have achieved top-class success at later ages. Therefore junior competitions can be seen as preparation for a later career: the junior competitor has to survive uninjured and with enthusiasm intact to pursue the sport at the highest levels.

If you are encouraging a child to do a particular sport, you must be aware and critical of your own motives. If you have in mind the money the child might earn as a successful sports professional, the possible honour and glory of winning medals, or the child's success where you have failed or did not have the opportunity, your motives are not necessarily geared to the child's best interests. The child should be free to make independent decisions about his or her career when he or she is old enough. These decisions may be made on the basis of opportunities you have provided, but the child should not be pressurized to make choices solely according to your criteria.

Sport and exercise for children should always be based on the principles of healthy body development. This applies equally to all organized sport for all age-groups, whether participation is at school, in clubs or at sports centres. Competition is only a small aspect of sport and exercise, and its problems in relation to children should not be allowed to obscure the wider significance of sport as a healthy recreational activity. All children and teenagers should be encouraged to do sports or exercise, and suitable fitness activities have to be devised for those who find the sporting disciplines too difficult. This is an essential requirement of modern physical education teaching in schools. To encourage children's participation in sport and exercise, and their subsequent pattern of healthy exercise throughout life, facilities and opportunities have to be widely available, and sports and different types of exercise have to be presented as fun.

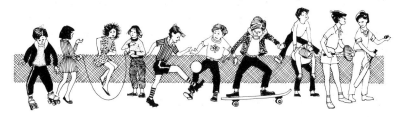

References

Introduction

1. Rutenfranz J 1986 Ethical considerations: the participation of children in elite sports. Paediatrician (Basel) 13 (1): 14–17

Chapter 1

1. Dubowitz L, Finnie N, Hyde S A, Scott O M, Vrbová G 1988 Improvement of muscle performance by chronic electrical stimulation in children with cerebral palsy. The Lancet 8585: 587–588
2. Jewell B 1977 Heritage of the Past: Sports and Games. Midas Books, Tunbridge Wells, Kent, p 5
3. Royal Canadian Airforce 1973 Physical Fitness. 5BX 11-minute-a-day plan for men. XBX 12-minute-a-day plan for women. Penguin Books, London
4. Riordan J 1981 The USSR. In: Riordan J (ed) Sport under Communism, 2nd edn. C. Hurst & Co, London, McGill-Queen's University Press, Montreal, pp 18–22
5. McIntosh P, Charlton V 1985 The Impact of Sport for All Policy 1966–1984 and a Way Forward. Sports Council, London
6. Ahonen J 1989 From Sports to Physiotherapy – and Back to Sports. In: Grisogono V A L (ed) I.P.P.T. Sports Injuries. Churchill Livingstone, Edinburgh, pp 110–115
7. Mason T 1988 Sport in Britain. Faber & Faber, London, pp 94–109
8. Tipton C M, Matthes R D, Maynard J A et al 1975 The influence of physical activity on ligaments and tendons. Medicine and Science in Sports and Exercise. 7: 165–175
9. Fentem P H, Bassey E J, Turnbull N B 1988 The New Case for Exercise. The Sports Council and the Health Education Authority, London
10. Vogel J A, Patton J F, Mello R P, Daniels W L 1986 An analysis of aerobic capacity in a large United States population. Journal of Applied Physiology 60: 494–500
11. Powell K E, Thompson P D, Caspersen C J, Kendrick J S 1987 Physical inactivity and the incidence of coronary heart disease. Annual Review of Public Health 8: 253–287

12. Schoutens A, Laurent E, Poortmans J R 1989 Effects of inactivity and exercise on bone. Sports Medicine 7: 71–81
13. School Sport Forum 1988 Sport and Young People: Partnership and Action. Sports Council, London, pp 14–15
14. Coe P 1986 Endurance Training and the Growing Child. In: Gleeson G (ed) The Growing Child in Competitive Sport. Hodder and Stoughton, London, pp 32–33
15. Riordan J 1987 Talent-Spotting, Ability Levels and Progress in Eastern Europe. Coaching Focus (National Coaching Foundation Magazine) 5: 2–3
16. Ahuja A, Ghosh A K 1989 Sports Physiotherapy in a sports institute in India. In: Grisogono V A L (ed) I.P.P.T. Sports Injuries. Churchill Livingstone, Edinburgh, pp 70–73
17. Purdam C R, Choquenot S, Colby J 1989 The physiotherapy unit at the Australian Institute of Sport. In: Grisogono V A L (ed) I.P.P.T. Sports Injuries. Churchill Livingstone, Edinburgh, pp 47–53
18. Martens R 1978 Joy and Sadness in Children's Sports. Human Kinetics Publishers Inc. Champaign, Illinois, pp 333–342
19. Smith J 1986 My Son Used to Enjoy Tennis . . . : A Concerned Parent's Perspective. In: Gleeson G (ed) The Growing Child in Competitive Sport. Hodder and Stoughton, London, pp 179–183
20. Buxton A 1989 Personal communication
21. Sceats A 1985 Sports and Leisure Club Management. Macdonald and Evans, Plymouth, pp 154–157
22. Rowley S 1986 The Role of the Parent in Youth Sport. In: Gleeson G (ed) The Growing Child in Competitive Sport. Hodder and Stoughton, London, pp 92–98
23. Rosen A 1978 Advice for Fathers. In: Martens R (ed) Joy and Sadness in Children's Sports. Human Kinetics Publishers Inc, Champaign, Illinois, pp 320–326
24. Martens R 1978 Problem Parents. In: Martens R (ed) Joy and Sadness in Children's Sports. Human Kinetics Publishers Inc, Champaign, Illinois, pp 333–342

Chapter 3

1. School Sport Forum 1988 Sport and Young People. Sports Council, London
2. American College of Sports Medicine 1988 Opinion Statement on Physical Fitness in Children and Youth. Medicine and Science in Sports and Exercise 20 (4): 422–423
3. Roberts R 1982 Marathon Running and Children. In: Russo P, Gass G, (eds) Children and Exercise, a Conference. Cumberland College of Health Sciences, Sydney, New South Wales, pp 51–55
4. Crasselt W 1988 Somatic development in children aged 7–18 years. In: Dirix A, Knuttgen H G, Tittel K (eds) The Olympic Book of Sports Medicine, Volume 1. Blackwell Scientific Publications, Oxford, pp 286–299

5. Scoles P V 1988 Pediatric Orthopedics in Clinical Practice, 2nd edn. Year Book Medical Publishers Inc., Chicago, pp 105, 184
6. Renström, P, Roux C 1988 Youth participation in sports. In: Dirix A, Knuttgen H G, Tittel K (eds) The Olympic Book of Sports Medicine, Volume 1. Blackwell Scientific Publications, Oxford, p 473
7. Anstiss T J 1990 Uses and abuses of drugs in sport: the athlete's view. In: Payne S D W (ed) Medicine, Sport and the Law. Blackwell Scientific Publications, Oxford, p 104
8. Benjamin I S 1990 The case against anabolic steroids. In: Payne S D W (ed) Medicine, Sport and the Law. Blackwell Scientific Publications, Oxford, pp 124–133
9. Leichter, I, Simkin A, Margulies J Y, Bivas A, Steinburg R, Giladi M, Milgrom C 1987 Bone formation in young adults – the effect of a short period of vigorous activity. In: Ruskin H, Simkin A (eds) Physical Fitness and the Ages of Man. Academon Press, Jerusalem, pp 218–234
10. Stewart M J 1981 Youth sport participation and the physiological functions of the child. Physical Educator 38 (2) 59–64
11. Anjos L A, Boileau R A 1988 Performance of undernourished and well nourished subjects in determinants of physical fitness tests. Revista Brasiliera de Ciencas e Movimento (Brazil) 2 (1): 21–29
12. Koethe R, Schmidt H 1984 Data for evaluation of the biological age of the vertebral column of trained adolescents and juniors. Sportorvosi Szemle/ Hungarian Review of Sports Medicine (Budapest) 25 (3): 173–186
13. Frisch R E 1984 Body fat, puberty and fertility. Biological Reviews (London) 59 (2): 161–188
14. Palgi Y, Gutin B, Young J, Alexandro D 1984 Physiological and anthropometric factors underlying endurance performance in children. International Journal of Sports Medicine (Stuttgart) 5 (2): 67–73
15. Johnson M L, Burke B S, Mayer J 1956 Relative importance of inactivity and overeating in the energy balance of obese high school girls. American Journal of Clinical Nutrition 4: 37–44
16. Rose H E, Mayer J 1968 Activity, calorie intake, fat storage and the energy balance of infants. Paediatrics 41: 18–28
17. Boileau R A, Lohman T G, Slaughter H 1985 Exercise and body composition of children and youth. Scandinavian Journal of Sports Science (Helsinki) 7 (1): 17–27
18. Highet R 1988 Athletic amenorrhoea: an update on aetiology, complications and management. Sports Medicine 7: 82–108
19. Välimäki I, Hursti M L, Pihlakoski L, Viikari J 1980 Exercise performance and serum lipids in relation to physical activity in schoolchildren. International Journal of Sports Medicine 1 (3): 132–136
20. Thorland W G, Gilliam T B 1981 Comparison of serum lipids between habitually low and high active pre-adolescent males. Medicine and Science in Sports and Exercise 13 (5): 316–321
21. Zonderland M L, Erich W B M, Peltenburg A L, Havekes L, Bernink M J E, Huisveld I A 1984 Apolipoprotein and lipid profiles in young

female athletes. International Journal of Sports Medicine 5 (2): 78–82

22. Máček M 1985 Indications and contraindications for sports in children and adolescents. International Council of Sports Science and Physical Education Review (Berlin) 8: 47–54

23. Potthast J, Klimt F 1988 Vertical power measurements of selected leg power exercises using capacitative measuring platforms. Deutsche Zeitschrift fur Sportmedizin (Cologne) 39 (8): 300–306

24. Nielsen B, Nielsen K, Behrendt-Hansen M, Asmussen E 1980 Training of functional muscle strength in girls 7–19 years old. In: Berg K, Erikson B (eds) Children and Exercise IX. University Park Press, Baltimore, pp 68–69

25. Pfeiffer R, Francis R S 1986 Effects of strength training on muscle development in pre-pubescent, pubescent and post-pubescent males. Physician and Sports Medicine 14: 134

26. Weltman A, Janney C, Rians C B, Strand K, Berg B, Tippit S, Wise J, Cahill B R, Katch F I 1986 The effects of hydraulic resistance strength training in pre-pubertal males. Medicine and Science in Sports and Exercise 18 (6): 629–638

27. Vrijens J 1978 Muscle strength development in the pre- and post-pubescent age group. Medicine and Sport (Basle) 11: 152

28. Bloomfield J, Blanksby B A, Ackland T R, Elliott B C 1985 The anatomical and physiological characteristics of pre-adolescent swimmers, tennis players and non-competitors. Australian Journal of Science and Medicine in Sport 17 (3): 19–23

29. American Academy of Pediatrics 1983 Weight training and weight lifting: information for the pediatrician. Physician and Sportsmedicine 11: 157

30. Bar-Or O 1988 Adaptability of the musculoskeletal, cardiovascular and respiratory systems. In: Dirix A, Knuttgen H G, Tittel K (eds) The Olympic Book of Sports Medicine, Volume 1. Blackwell Scientific Publications, Oxford, p 270

31. Reid D C 1983 The Young Athlete. In: Howell M L, Bullock M I (eds) Physiotherapy in Sport. University of Queensland, Department of Human Movement Studies, pp 9–15

32. Bar-Or O 1985 Methodological considerations in pediatric physiology. In: Russo P, Gass G (eds) Children and Exercise: Proceedings of 5th Biennial Conference. Cumberland College of Health Sciences, Sydney, New South Wales, pp 105–115

33. Nakao M, Inoue Y, Matsuhita K, Murakami H 1986 Simple methods for measuring leg muscular endurance. Journal of Sports Medicine and Physical Fitness (Turin) 26 (3): 285–291

34. Kurouski T T 1983 Anaerobic power of children from age 9 through 15 years. MSc Thesis, 1977, Florida State University. In: Bar-Or O (ed) Pediatric Sports Medicine, Springer-Verlag, New York, pp 11–12

35. Bar-Or O 1983 Pediatric Sports Medicine. Springer-Verlag, New York, a) p 13, b) 32, c) 262–263, d) 276–277, e) 281

36. Inbar O, Bar-Or O 1986 Anaerobic characteristics in male children and

adolescents. Medicine and Science in Sports and Exercise 18 (3): 264–269
37. Eriksson B O, Karlsson J, Saltin B 1971 Muscle metabolites during exercise in pre-pubertal boys. Acta Paediatrica Scandinavica (Supplement) 217: 154–157
38. Simon G, Berg A, Dickhuth H H, Simon-Alt A, Keul J 1981 Determination of the anaerobic threshold depending on age and performance potential. Deutsche Zeitschrift fuer Sportmedizin 32: 7–10
39. Canbaz M, Gokhan N, Yenson M 1981 Blood lactate levels of judo-karate trained and nontrained children in maximal and supramaximal exercise. Turkish Journal of Sports Medicine 16 (3): 91–93
40. Krahenbuhl G S, Pangrazi R P 1983 Characteristics associated with running performance in young boys. Medicine and Science in Sports and Exercise 15 (6): 486–490
41. Rotstein A, Dotan R, Bar-Or O, Tenenbaum G 1986 Effect of training on anaerobic threshold, maximal power and anaerobic performance of preadolescent boys. International Journal of Sports Medicine 7 (5): 281–286
42. Andersen K L, Rutenfranz J, Ilmarinen J, Berndt I, Kylian H, Ruppel M, Seliger V 1983 The growth of lung volumes affected by physical performance capacity in boys and girls during adolescence and childhood. European Journal of Applied Physiology and Occupational Physiology 52 (4): 380–384
43. Wanne O P S, Haapoja E 1988 Blood pressure during exercise in healthy children. European Journal of Applied Physiology and Occupational Physiology 58 (1/2): 62–67
44. Michel-Panichi C, Mandel C, Auriacombe L, Pedroni E, Kachaner J, Hennequet A 1987 Echocardiography in children practising ice skating. Médecine du Sport (Paris) 61 (3): 159–163
45. Morganroth J, Maron B J, Henry W L, Epstein E E 1975 Comparative left ventricular dimensions in trained athletes. Annals of International Medicine 88: 521
46. Vollmer-Larsen A, Vollmer-Larsen B, Godtfredsen J 1987 Alterations in the shape and size of the heart resulting from training. Ugeskrift for Laeger (Copenhagen) 149 (22): 1447–1450
47. Shapiro L (Consultant Cardiologist, Papworth Hospital, England) 1989 Personal communication
48. Hanne-Paparo N 1987 The athlete's heart: a review. International Journal of Sports Cardiology (Turin) 4 (1): 47–57
49. Nuviala R J, Giner M A, Lapieza M G 1987 Comparative study of recovery ECG after an aerobic cycle ergometer test and the Wingate test in children. Kinésiologie (Paris) 26 (111): 7–13
50. Deng S, Huang R, Sun A, 1984 The relationship between stroke volume and heart rate during graded exercise in children. Chinese Journal of Sports Medicine (Beijing) 3 (1): 16–22
51. Tanner J M 1949 Fallacy of per-weight and per-surface-area standards

and their relation to spurious correlation. Journal of Applied Physiology 2: 1–15

52. Winter E 1990 Personal communication. Department of Sports Science, Bedford College of Higher Education, Bedford, England

53. Sharp N C C 1983 Fitness testing for racket players. In: Proceedings of the 3rd Guinness Conference on Sport. Northern Ireland Institute of Coaching, pp 56–62

54. Armstrong N 1989 Field testing children's physical fitness. In: Cooke G (ed) The Growing Child in Competitive Sport. Proceedings of the 1989 BISC/Adidas International Congress. British Institute of Sports Coaches, Leeds, pp 97–102

55. Armstrong N, Balding J, Gentle P, Kirby B 1990 Estimation of risk factors for chronic disease in children from 15 countries. Preventive Medicine 10: 121–132

56. Anderson L B, Henckel P, Saltin B 1987 Maximal oxygen uptake in Danish adolescents 16–19 years of age. European Journal of Applied Physiology and Occupational Physiology 56 (1): 74–82

57. Saris W H M, de-Koning F, Elvers J W H, de Boo T, Binkhorst R A 1984 Estimation of W170 and maximal oxygen consumption in young children by different treadmill tests. In: Ilmarinen J, Välimäki I (eds) Children and Sport: Paediatric Work Physiology. Springer-Verlag, Berlin

58. Saris W H M, Noordeloos A M, Ringnalda B E M, Van't-Hof M A, Binkhorst R A 1985 Reference values for aerobic power of healthy 4- to 18-year-old Dutch children: preliminary results. In: Binkhorst R A (ed) Children and Exercise XI. Human Kinetics Publishers, Illinois, pp 151–160

59. Sheehan J M, Rowland T W, Burke E J 1987 A comparison of four treadmill protocols for determination of maximum oxygen uptake in 10- to 12-year-old boys. International Journal of Sports Medicine (Stuttgart) 8 (1): 31–34

60. Davies C T M 1982 Aerobic performance in young children. In: Russo P F, Gass G (eds) Children and Exercise, a Conference. Cumberland College of Health Sciences, Sydney, New South Wales, pp 42–45

61. Leger L A, Mercier D, Gadoury C, Lambert J 1988 The Multistage 20 metre shuttle run test for aerobic fitness. British Journal of Sports Science (London) 6 (2): 93–101

62. van-Mechelen W, Hlobil H, Kemper H C G 1986 Validation of two running tests as estimates of maximal aerobic power in children. European Journal of Applied Physiology and Occupational Physiology 55 (5): 503–506

63. Faulman L 1990 Personal communication from unpublished work in progress. British Olympic Medical Centre, Northwick Park Hospital and Clinical Research Centre, London

64. Eston R G, Brodie D A 1985 The assessment of maximal oxygen uptake from running tests. Physical Education Review (North Humberside, England) 8 (1): 26–34

65. Gaisl G, Buchberger J 1980 Determination of the aerobic and anaerobic thresholds of 10–11-year-old boys using blood gas analysis. In: Berg K, Eriksson B O (eds) Children and Exercise IX. University Park Press, Baltimore, pp 93–98

66. Gaisl, G, Weisspeiner G 1988 A noninvasive method of determining the anaerobic threshold in children. International Journal of Sports Medicine (Stuttgart) 9 (1): 41–44

67. Haffor A A, Kirk P A C 1988 Anaerobic threshold and relation of ventilation to CO_2 output during exercise in 11-year-olds. Journal of Sports Medicine and Physical Fitness (Turin) 28 (1): 74–78

68. Reybrouck T, Weymans M, Stijns H, Knops J, van-der-Hauwert L 1985 Ventilatory anaerobic threshold in healthy children. Age and sex differences. European Journal of Applied Physiology and Occupational Physiology 54 (3): 278–284

69. Cooper D M 1985 Gas exchange kinetics at the onset of exercise during growth in children. Scandinavian Journal of Sports Science (Helsinki) 7 (1): 3–9

70. Morris J N, Clayton D G, Everitt M G, Semmence A M, Burgess E H 1990 Exercise in leisure time: coronary attack and death rates. British Heart Journal 63: 325–334

71. Becker D M, Vaccaro P 1983 Anaerobic threshold alterations caused by endurance training in young children. Journal of Sports Medicine and Physical Fitness (Turin) 23 (4): 445–449

72. Atomi Y, Iwaoka K, Hatta H, Miyashita M, Yamamoto Y 1986 Daily physical activity levels in preadolescent boys related to VO2 max and lactate thresholds. European Journal of Applied Physiology and Occupational Physiology 55 (2): 151–161

73. Letzelter M 1987 The quantity law of practice in physical education: the dependence of achievement progress on the initial ability level. Sportunterricht (Schorndorf, FRG) 36 (2): 42–54

74. Krahenbuhl G S, Skinner J S, Kohrt W M 1985 Developmental aspects of maximal aerobic power in children. Exercise and Sport Science Review (New York) 13: 503–538

75. Rusko H 1985 Youth and top-class sport: endurance training effects on young athletes. International Council of Sports Science and Physical Education Review (Berlin) 8: 54–64

76. Kofsky P R, Goode R C, Romet T T 1983 Effects of a short period of intense activity on school children. Australian Journal of Sports Science 3 (1): 19–21

77. Rowland T W 1985 Aerobic response to endurance training in prepubescent children: a critical analysis. Medicine and Science in Sports and Exercise (Indianapolis) 17 (5): 493–497

78. Kemper H C G 1983 Physiological aspects of endurance sport in young people. International Journal of Physical Education 20 (4): 22–27

79. Buzina R, Grgić Z, Jusić M, Sapunar J, Milanović N, Brubacher G 1982

Nutritional status and physical working capacity. Clinical Nutrition 36 (6): 429–438

80. Cooke C B 1990 Running efficiency: a biomechanical and physiological evaluation of normal and loaded horizontal running. PhD Thesis. University of Birmingham, England

81. Åstrand P-O 1952 Experimental studies of physical working capacity in relation to sex and age. Copenhagen Munksgaard

82. Skinner J S, Bar-Or O, Bergsteinova V 1971 Comparison of continuous and intermittent tests for determining maximal oxygen intake in children. Acta Paediatrica Scandinavica Supplement 217: 24–28

83. Rowland T W, Auchinachie J A, Keenan T J, Green G M 1988 Submaximal running economy and treadmill performance in prepubertal boys. International Journal of Sports Medicine (Stuttgart) 9 (3): 201–204

84. Burkett L N, Fernhall B, Walters S C 1985 Physiological effects of distance running on teenage females. Research Quarterly for Exercise and Sports 56: 215

85. Villagra F 1989 The storage of elastic energy in repetitive movement. MSc Thesis, University of Birmingham, England

86. Alexander R McN 1987 The spring in your step. New Scientist 114: 42–44

87. MacDougal J D, Roche P D, Bar-Or O, Moroz J R 1983 Maximum aerobic capacity of Canadian schoolchildren: prediction based on age-related cost of running. International Journal of Sports Medicine 4: 194–198

88. Hebbelinck M 1988 Flexibility. In: Dirix A, Knuttgen H G, Tittel K (eds) The Olympic Book of Sports Medicine, Volume 1. Blackwell Scientific Publications, Oxford, pp 212–217

89. O'Neill D B, Micheli L J 1988 Overuse injuries in the young athlete. Clinics in Sports Medicine 7 (3): 591–610

90. Highgenboten C L 1981 Children's knee problems. Orthopedic Review 10: 37–48

91. Beck J L, Day R W 1985 Overuse injuries. Clinics in Sports Medicine 4 (3): 553–573

92. Safran M R, Garrett W E, Seaber A V, Glisson R R, Ribbeck B M 1988 The role of warm-up in muscular injury prevention. American Journal of Sports Medicine 16 (2): 123–129

93. Ekstrand J, Gillquist J 1983 The avoidability of soccer injuries. International Journal of Sports Medicine 4: 124–128

94. Wiktorsson-Moller M, Oberg B, Ekstrand J, Gillquist J 1983 Effects of warming up, massage, and stretching on range of motion and muscle strength in the lower extremity. American Journal of Sports Medicine 11 (4): 249–252

95. Wallace L A, Mangine R E, Malone T 1985 The knee. In: Gould J A, Davies G J (eds) Orthopaedic and Sports physical therapy. C V Mosby Company, St. Louis, p 351

222 Children and Sport

96. Feiring D C, Derscheid G L 1989 The role of preseason conditioning in preventing athletic injuries. Clinics in Sports Medicine 8 (3): 361–372
97. Safran M R, Seaber A V, Garrett W E 1989 Warm-up and muscular injury prevention: an update. Sports Medicine 8 (4): 239–249
98. Kulund D N, Tottossy M 1983 Warm up, strength and power. Orthopedic Clinics of North America 14 (2): 427–448
99. Zachazewski J E, Reischl S 1986 Flexibility for the runner: Specific program considerations. Topics in Acute Care in Trauma and Rehabilitation 1: 9–27
100. Arens D 1983 Train or play for the young runner: a study of specialisation versus general development for the young. Australian Track and Field Coaches' Association, Sydney
101. Araki T, Toda Y, Matsushita K, Tsujino A 1979 Age differences in sweating during muscular exercise. Japanese Journal of Physical Fitness and Sports Medicine 28: 239–248
102. Davies C T M 1982 The thermal stress of prolonged exercise in children. In: Russo P F, Gass G (eds) Children and Exercise, A Conference. Cumberland College of Health Sciences, New South Wales, Sydney, pp 38–41
103. Máčková J, Sturmova M, Máček M 1984 Prolonged exercise in prepubertal boys in warm and cold environments. In: Ilmarinen J, Välimäki I (eds) Children and Sport: Paediatric Work Physiology. Springer-Verlag, Berlin, pp 135–141
104. Sloan R E G, Keatinge W R 1973 Cooling rates of young people swimming in cold water. Journal of Applied Physiology 41: 233–245
105. Craig A B 1983 Temperature regulation and immersion. In: Hollander (ed) Biomechanics and Medicine in Swimming: Proceedings of the Fourth International Symposium of Biomechanics in Swimming and the Fifth International Congress on Swimming Medicine. Human Kinetics Publishers, Champaign, Illinois, pp 263–274
106. Haymes E M, McCormick R J, Buskirk E R 1975 Heat tolerance of exercising lean and obese prepubertal boys. Journal of Applied Physiology 39: 457–461
107. Bar-Or O, Dotan R, Inbar O 1980 Voluntary hypohydration in 10- to 12-year-old boys. Journal of Applied Physiology 48: 104–108
108. Davies C T M, Fohlin L, Thoren C 1980 Perception of exertion in anorexia nervosa patients. In: Berg K, Eriksson B O (eds) Children and Exercise IX. University Park Press, Baltimore, Maryland, pp 327–332
109. Bar-Or O 1977 Age-related changes in exercise perception. In: Borg G (ed) Physical Work and Effort. Pergamon Press, Oxford, pp 256–265
110. Máček M, Vávra J, Mrzena B 1971 Intermittent exercise of supramaximal intensity in children. Acta Paediatrica Scandinavica 217: 29
111. Mészáros J, Mohácsi J, Frenkl R, Szabó T, Smodis J 1986 Age dependency in the development of motor-test performance. In: Rutenfranz J, Mocellin R, Klimt F (eds) Children and Exercise XII. Human Kinetics Publishers, Champaign, Illinois, pp 347–354

112. Schmucker B, Rigauer B, Hinrichs W, Trawinski J 1984 Motor abilities and habitual physical activity in children. In: Ilmarinen J, Välimäki I (eds) Children and Sport. Springer-Verlag, Berlin, pp 46–52
113. Máček M, Vávra J 1981 Prolonged exercise in 14-year-old girls. International Journal of Sports Medicine 2: 228
114. Máček M 1988 Training Children and Adolescents: Age and General Development. In: Dirix A, Knuttgen H G, Tittel K (eds) The Olympic Book of Sports Medicine, Volume 1. Blackwell Scientific Publications, Oxford, pp. 301, 305, 304

Chapter 4

1. Layzer R B 1986 Muscle Pain, Cramps and Fatigue. In: Engel A G, Banker B Q (eds) Myology, Basic and Clinical. McGraw-Hill Book Co., New York, p 1910
2. Castellanos J, Axelrod D 1990 Effect of habitual knuckle cracking on hand function. Annals of the Rheumatic Diseases 49 (5): 308–309
3. Zaricznyj B, Shattuck J M, Mast T A, Robertson R V, D'Elia G 1980 Sports-related injuries in school-aged children. American Journal of Sports Medicine 8 (5): 318–324
4. Rutherford G W, Miles R B, Brown V R, MacDonald B 1981 Overview of sports-related injuries to persons 5–14 years of age. United States Consumer Product Safety Commission, Washington, DC, iv: 47
5. Mueller F, Blyth C 1982 Epidemiology of sports injuries in children. Clinics in Sports Medicine 1 (3): 343–352
6. Latinis B 1983 Frequent Sports Injuries of Children: Etiology, Treatment and Prevention. Issues of Comprehensive Pediatric Nursing (Washington) 6 (3): 167–178
7. Micheli L J 1984 Sports Injuries in the Young Athlete: Questions and Controversies. In: Micheli L J (ed) Pediatric and Adolescent Sports Medicine. Little, Brown and Company, Boston, p 6
8. MacDonald G L 1985 Sports Injuries in Children. Necessary Consequence of Competition? Postgraduate Medicine (Minneapolis) 78 (1): 279–281, 284–5, 289
9. Micheli L J 1986 Pediatric and Adolescent Sports Injuries: Recent Trends. Exercise and Sport Sciences Reviews (New York) 14: 359–374
10. Tursz, A, Crost M 1986 Sport-related injuries in children: a study of their characteristics, frequency and severity, with comparison to other types of accidental injuries. American Journal of Sports Medicine 14 (4): 294–299
11. Backx F J, Erich W B, Kemper A B, Verbeek A L 1989 Sports injuries in school-age children. An epidemiologic study. American Journal of Sports Medicine 17 (2): 234–240
12. Lysens R J, Ostyn M S, Vanden Auweele Y, Lefevre J, Vuylsteke M, Renson L 1989 The accident-prone and overuse-prone profiles of the young athlete. American Journal of Sports Medicine 17 (5): 612–619
13. Kvist, M, Kujala U M, Heinonen O J, Vuori I V, Aho A J, Pajulo O, Hintsa

A, Parvinen T 1989 Sports-related injuries in children. International Journal of Sports Medicine 10 (2): 81–86

14. Sahlin Y 1990 Sport accidents in childhood. British Journal of Sports Medicine 24 (1): 40–44
15. Horne J, Cockshott W P, Shannon H S 1987 Spinal column damage from water ski jumping. Skeletal Radiology 16 (8): 612–616
16. Nudel D B, Bassett I, Gurian A, Diamant S, Weinhouse E, Gootman N 1989 Young long distance runners. Physiological and psychological characteristics. Clinics in Pediatrics (Philadelphia) 28 (11): 500–505
17. Grisogono V A L 1981 The Injuries Service at the Crystal Palace. British Journal of Sports Medicine 15 (1): 39–43
18. Grisogono V A L 1986 Prevention and Prophylaxis, In: Helal B, King J B, Grange W J (eds) Sports Injuries and their Treatment. Chapman and Hall Medical, London, p 4
19. Pavlov H 1990 Athletic injuries. Radiologic Clinics of North America (Philadelphia) 28 (2): 435–443
20. Graham G P, Fairclough J A 1988 Early osteoarthritis in young sportsmen with severe anterolateral instability of the knee. Injury 19 (4): 247–248
21. McBride I D, Reid J G 1988 Biomechanical considerations of the menisci of the knee. Canadian Journal of Applied Sports Sciences 13 (4): 175–187.
22. Felson D T 1988 Epidemiology of hip and knee osteoarthritis. Epidemiologic Review 10: 1–28
23. Hougaard K, Thomsen P B, 1989 Traumatic hip dislocation in children. Follow up of 13 cases. Orthopedics 12 (3): 375–378
24. Murray R O, Duncan C 1971 Athletic activity in adolescence as an etiologic factor in degenerative hip disease. Journal of Bone and Joint Surgery 53B: 406–419
25. Neusel E, Arza D, Rompe G, Steinbruck K 1987 (long-term roentgenologic studies in peak performance javelin throwers) (article in German) Sportverletzung Sportschaden 1 (2): 76–80
26. Panush R S, Brown D G 1987 Exercise and arthritis. Sports Medicine 4 (1): 54–64
27. Knight K L 1985 Cryotherapy: Theory, Technique and Physiology. Chattanooga Corporation Educational Division, Tennessee, pp 53–54
28. Roy S, Irvin R 1983 Sports Medicine. Prevention, Evaluation, Management and Rehabilitation. Prentice-Hall Inc., New Jersey, pp 78–93
29. Coady C, Stanish W D 1988 Emergencies in Sports: The Young Athlete. Clinics in Sports Medicine 7 (3): 625–640

Chapter 6

1. Scoles P V 1988 Pediatric Orthopedics in Clinical Practice. 2nd edn. Year Book Medical Publishers Inc., Chicago, pp 1–22
2. Armstrong N 1989 Field Testing Children's Physical Fitness. In: Cooke G (ed) The Growing Child in Competitive Sport. Proceedings of the 1989 BISC/Adidas International Congress. British Institute of Sports Coaches, Leeds

3. Council of Europe Committee for the Development of Sport 1988 EUROFIT. Handbook for the EUROFIT Tests of Physical Fitness. Sports Council, London

4. Marshall J L, Tischler H M 1978 Screening for Sports, Guidelines. New York Journal of Medicine, 78: 243

5. Blackburn Jr T A (ed) 1979 Guidelines for Pre-Season Athletic Participation Evaluation. Sports Medicine Section of the American Physical Therapists' Association, Columbus, Georgia

6. Kulund D N 1982 The Injured Athlete. J B Lippincott Company, Philadelphia, pp 5–23

7. Roy S, Irvin R 1983 Sports Medicine. Prevention, Evaluation, Management and Rehabilitation. Prentice-Hall Inc, New Jersey, pp. 11–27

8. Micheli L J, Yost J G 1984 Preparticipation Evaluation and First Aid for Sports. In: Micheli L J (ed) Pediatric and Adolescent Sports Medicine. Little, Brown and Company, Boston/Toronto, pp 30–39

9. Eggart J S, Leigh D, Vergamini G 1985 Preseason Athletic Physical Evaluation. In: Gould J A, Davies G J (eds) Orthopaedic and Sports physical therapy. C V Mosby Company, St. Louis, pp 605–642

10. Kibler W B, Chandler T J, Uhl T, Maddux R E 1989 A musculoskeletal approach to the preparticipation physical examination. American Journal of Sports Medicine 17 (4): 525–531

11. Linder C W 1989 The Preparticipation Health Evaluation of High School Athletes. In: Smith N J (ed) Common Problems in Pediatric Sports Medicine, Year Book Medical Publishers, Inc, Chicago, pp 358–366

12. Rooks D S, Micheli L J 1988 Musculoskeletal Assessment and Training: The Young Athlete. Clinics in Sports Medicine 7 (3): 641

13. Preece M 1989 Growth, Development and Youth Sport. In: Cooke G (ed) The Growing Child in Competitive Sport. Proceedings of the 1989 BISC/Adidas International Congress. British Institute of Sports Coaches, Leeds, pp 2–6; 17–20

14. Hodgson D 1989 Good Behaviour, Great Performance. In: Cooke G (ed). Op. cit. pp 34–41

15. Rowley S 1989 Intensive Training and its Effect on Family Life. In: Cooke G (ed). Op. cit. pp 50–56

16. Graham P 1989 Retiring from Youth Sport, Turbulence or Tranquillity. In: Cooke G (ed). Op. cit. pp 77–80

17. Maffuli N, Helms P 1989 Sports Injuries in Intensively Trained Children. In: Cooke G (ed.) Op. cit. pp 81–88

18. Grisogono V A L 1984 Sports Injuries, A Self-Help Guide. John Murray, London

Chapter 7

1. Williams P L, Warwick R, Dyson M, Bannister L H (eds) Gray's Anatomy, 37th edn. Churchill Livingstone, Edinburgh, pp 269–312

2. Reigger C L 1985 Mechanical properties of bone. In: Gould J A, Davies

G J (eds) Orthopaedic and Sports physical therapy. C V Mosby Co., St. Louis

3. Scoles P V 1988 Pediatric Orthopedics in Clinical Practice, 2nd edn. Year Book Medical Publishers Inc., Chicago, p 29

4. Weber B G, Brunner C, Freuler F (eds) 1980 Treatment of Fractures in Children and Adolescents. Springer-Verlag, Berlin

5. Pappas A M 1983 Epiphyseal injuries in sports. Physician and Sportsmedicine 11 (6): 140–148

6. Larson R L 1973 Epiphyseal injuries in the adolescent athlete. Orthopedic Clinics of North America 4: 839–851

7. Wenger D R 1984 Slipped Capital Femoral Epiphysis. In: Tronzo R G (ed) Surgery of the Hip Joint. Springer-Verlag, New York

8. Roberts J 1979 Osteochondritis dissecans. In: Kennedy J C (ed) The Injured Adolescent Knee. Williams & Wilkins, Baltimore

9. Hughston J, Hergenroeder P, Courtenay B 1984 Osteochondritis dissecans of the femoral condyle. Journal of Bone and Joint Surgery 66A: 323–329

10. McManama G B 1988 Ankle Injuries in the Young Athlete. Clinics in Sports Medicine 7 (3): 547–562

11. Coady C, Stanish W D 1988 Emergencies in Sports: The Young Athlete. Clinics in Sports Medicine 7 (3): 625–639

12. Salter R B, Harris W R 1963 Injuries involving the epiphyseal plate. Journal of Bone and Joint Surgery 45A: 587

13. Devas M 1963 Stress fractures in children. Journal of Bone and Joint Surgery 45B: 528–541

14. Devas M 1975 Stress Fractures. Churchill Livingstone, Edinburgh, p 5

15. Smith A D 1988 Children and Sports. In: Scoles P V Pediatric Orthopedics in Clinical Practice, 2nd edn. Year Book Medical Publishers Inc., Chicago, p 275

16. Rossi F 1978 Spondylolysis, spondylolisthesis and sport. Journal of Sports Medicine and Physical Fitness 18 (4): 317–340

17. Colby, J, Fricker P 1984 Can we prevent back injuries to elite women gymnasts? Sports Science and Medicine Quarterly 1 (1): 13–16

18. Hoshina H 1980 Spondylolysis in athletes. Physician and Sportsmedicine 8 (9): 75–77

19. Micheli L J, Hall J E, Miller M E 1980 Use of modified Boston brace for back injuries in athletes. American Journal of Sports Medicine 8 (5): 351–356

20. Blackburne J S, Velikas E P 1977 Spondylolisthesis in children and adolescents. Journal of Bone and Joint Surgery 59B: 490–494

21. Bell D F, Ehrlich M G, Zaleske D J 1988 Brace treatment for symptomatic spondylolisthesis. Clinical Orthopaedics and Related Research 236: 192–198

22. Roy S, Irvin R 1983 Sports Medicine. Prevention, Evaluation, Management, and Rehabilitation. Prentice-Hall Inc., New Jersey, p 138

23. Commandré F A, Argenson C, Bouzayen A, Vanuxem P, Zakarian H 1988 Principles of diagnosis and management of traumatic injuries. In: Dirix A,

Knuttgen H G, Tittel K (eds) The Olympic Book of Sports Medicine, Volume 1. Blackwell Scientific Publications, Oxford, pp 403–405

24. Micheli L J 1987 The traction apophysitises. Clinics in Sports Medicine 6 (2): 389–404
25. Kujala U M, Kvist M, Heinonen O 1985 Osgood-Schlatter's disease in adolescent athletes. A retrospective study of incidence and duration. American Journal of Sports Medicine 13 (4): 237–241
26. Clancy W G, Foltz A S 1976 Iliac apophysitis in stress fractures in adolescent runners. American Journal of Sports Medicine 4: 214–218
27. Dyson M 1989 The Use of Ultrasound in Sports Physiotherapy. In: Grisogono V A L (ed) International Perspectives in Physical Therapy, Sports Injuries. Churchill Livingstone, Edinburgh, p 228
28. Mirbey J, Besancenot J, Chambers R T, Durey A, Vichard P 1988 Avulsion fractures of the tibial tuberosity in the adolescent athlete. American Journal of Sports Medicine 16 (4): 336–340

Useful reading

Adams J E 1968 Bone injuries in very young athletes. Clinical Orthopaedics and Related Research 58: 129–140
Cahill B 1985 Treatment of Juvenile Osteochondritis Dissecans and Osteochondritis Dissecans of the Knee. Clinics in Sports Medicine 4: 367–384
Cantu R C 1988 Head and Spine Injuries in the Young Athlete. Clinics in Sports Medicine 7 (3): 459–472
Clain M R, Harshman E B 1989 Overuse injuries in children and adolescents. Physician and Sportsmedicine 17 (9): 111–123
Ichikawa N, Ohara Y, Morishita T, Taniguichi Y, Koshikawa A, Matsukura N 1982 Aetiological study on spondylolysis from a biomechanical aspect. British Journal of Sports Medicine 16 (3): 135–141
Ireland M L, Andrews J R 1988 Shoulder and Elbow Injuries in the Young Athlete. Clinics in Sports Medicine 7 (3): 473–493
Letts M, Smallman T, Afanasiev R, Gouw G 1986 Fracture of the pars interarticularis in adolescent athletes: a clinical-biomechanical analysis. Journal of Pediatric Orthopedics 6 (1): 40–46
Torg J S 1985 Epidemiology, Pathomechanics, and Prevention of Athletic Injuries to the Cervical Spine. Medicine and Science in Sports and Exercise 17: 295
Walter N E, Wolf M D 1977 Stress fractures in young athletes. American Journal of Sports Medicine 5 (4): 165–170
Waters P M, Millis M B 1988 Hip and Pelvic Injuries in the Young Athlete. Clinics in Sports Medicine 7 (3): 513–525

Chapter 8

1. Scoles P V 1988 Pediatric Orthopedics in Clinical Practice, 2nd edn. Year Book Medical Publishers Inc., Chicago, p 105

2. Webber A 1988 Acute Soft-Tissue Injuries in the Young Athlete. Clinics in Sports Medicine 7 (3): 611–624
3. O'Neill D B, Micheli L J 1988 Overuse Injuries in the Young Athlete. Clinics in Sports Medicine 7 (3): 591–610
4. Santopietro F J 1988 Foot and Foot-Related Injuries in the Young Athlete. Clinics in Sports Medicine 7 (3): 563–589
5. McManama G B 1988 Ankle Injuries in the Young Athlete. Clinics in Sports Medicine 7 (3): 547–562
6. Garrick J G, Requa R K 1973 Role of External Support in the Prevention of Ankle Sprains. Medicine and Science in Sports 5: 200–203
7. Firer P 1990 Effectiveness of taping for the prevention of ankle ligament sprains. British Journal of Sports Medicine 24 (1): 47–50
8. Grisogono V A L 1989 Physiotherapy Treatment for Achilles Tendon Injuries. Physiotherapy 75 (10): 562–572
9. Black K P, Schultz T K, Cheung N L 1990 Compartment syndromes in athletes. Clinics in Sports Medicine 9 (2): 471–487
10. Scoles P V 1988 Pediatric Orthopedics in Clinical Practice, 2nd edn. Year Book Medical Publishers Inc., Chicago, pp 93–103
11. Smillie I S 1978 Injuries of the Knee Joint, 5th edn. Churchill Livingstone, Edinburgh, p 16
12. Grisogono V A L 1984 Sports Injuries, A Self-help Guide. John Murray, London, pp 132–135
13. Garrett W E, Califf J C, Bassett F H 1984 Histochemical correlates of hamstring injuries. American Journal of Sports Medicine 12 (2): 98–103
14. Kulund D N 1982 The injured athlete. J B Lippincott Co, Philadelphia, p 358
15. Waters P M, Millis M B 1988 Hip and Pelvic Injuries in the Young Athlete. Clinics in Sports Medicine 7 (3): 513–525
16. Lorenzton R 1988 Causes of injuries: intrinsic factors. In: Dirix A, Knuttgen H G, Tittel K (eds) The Olympic Book of Sports Medicine, Volume I. Blackwell Scientific Publications, Oxford, pp 384–385
17. Ohlen G, Wredmark T, Spangfort E 1989 Spinal sagittal configuration and mobility related to low-back pain in the female gymnast. Spine 14 (8): 847–861
18. Oseid S et al 1984 Prevention of lower back pain in young female gymnasts. In: Bachl N, Prokop L, Suckert R (eds) Current Topics in Sports Medicine (Report of the World Congress, 1982, Vienna), Urban abd Schwarzenberg, Vienna
19. Horne J, Cockshot W P, Shannon H S 1987 Spinal column damage from water ski jumping. Skeletal Radiology 16 (8): 612–616
20. Czorny A, Forlodou P, Kilic K, Auque J, Hepner H 1988 (Lumbar disc hernia in children. Apropos of 12 cases.) (Article in French.) Neurochirurgie 34 (6): 389–393
21. Ireland M L, Andrews J R 1988 Shoulder and elbow injuries in the young athlete. Clinics in Sports Medicine 7 (3): 473–494

22. Chandler T J, Kibler W B, Uhl T L, Wooten B, Kiser A, Stone E 1990 Flexibility comparisons of junior elite tennis players to other athletes. American Journal of Sports Medicine 18 (2): 134–136

23. Greipp J 1985 Swimmer's Shoulder – the influence of flexibility and weight training. Physician and Sports Medicine 13: 92–105

24. Newberg A H 1987 The radiographic evaluation of shoulder and elbow pain in the athlete. Clinics in Sports Medicine 6 (4): 785–809

25. Pappas A M 1982 Elbow problems associated with baseball during childhood and adolescence. Clinical Orthopaedics and Related Research 164: 30–41

26. Scoles P V 1988 Pediatric Orthopedics in Clinical Practice, 2nd edn. Year Book Medical Publishers Inc., Chicago, pp 40–43

27. Simmons B P, Lovallo J L 1988 Hand and wrist injuries in children. Clinics in Sports Medicine 7 (3): 495–512

28. Daly P J, Sim F H, Simonet W T 1990 Ice hockey injuries: a review. Sports Medicine 10 (2): 122–123

29. McCue F C, Mayer V 1989 Rehabilitation of common athletic injuries of the hand and wrist. Clinics in Sports Medicine 8 (4): 731–776

Chapter 9

1. Nisonson B 1989 Acute Hemarthrosis of the Adolescent Knee. Physician and Sportsmedicine 17 (4): 75–87

2. Smillie I S 1978 Injuries of the Knee Joint, 5th edn. Churchill Livingstone, Edinburgh, pp 99; 5–12; 10

3. Macnicol M F 1986 The Problem Knee: Diagnosis and Management in the Younger Patient. William Heinemann Medical Books, London, pp 73–79, 84–97

4. Steiner M E, Grana W A 1988 The Young Athlete's Knee: Recent Advances. Clinics in Sports Medicine 7 (3): 527–545

5. Angel K R, Hall D J 1989 Anterior cruciate ligament injury in children and adolescents. Arthroscopy 5 (3): 192–196

6. Frank C, Strother R 1989 Isolated Posterior Cruciate Ligament Injury in a Child: Literature Review and a Case Report. Canadian Journal of Surgery 32 (5): 373–374

7. Grisogono V A L 1988 Knee Health: Problems, Prevention and Cure. John Murray, London, pp 27, 104

8. Bradley G, Shives T, Samuelson K 1979 Ligament injuries in the knees of children. Journal of Bone and Joint Surgery 61A: 588–591

9. Micheli L, Slater J, Woods E, et al 1986 Patella alta and the adolescent growth spurt. Clinical Orthopaedics and Related Research. 213: 159–162

10. Smith A D, Scoles P V 1988 The Knee. In: Scoles P V Pediatric Orthopedics in Clinical Practice, 2nd edn. Year Book Medical Publishers Inc., Chicago, p 134

11. Beckman M, Craig R, Lehman R C 1989 Rehabilitation of Patellofemoral Dysfunction in the Athlete. Clinics in Sports Medicine 8 (4): 841–860

12. McConnell J 1986 The Management of Chondromalacia Patellae: A Long Term Solution. Australian Journal of Physiotherapy 32 (4): 215–223

Chapter 11

1. Department of Health and Social Security, Committee on Medical Aspects of Food Policy 1979 Recommended Daily Amount of Food Energy and Nutrients for Groups of People in the United Kingdom. Report on Health and Social Subjects No. 15. Her Majesty's Stationery Office, London
2. Department of Health and Social Security, Committee on Medical Aspects of Food Policy 1984 Diet and Cardiovascular Disease. Report on Health and Social Subjects No. 28. Her Majesty's Stationery Office, London
3. Department of Health and Social Security, Committee on Medical Aspects of Food Policy 1989 Present Day Practice in Infant Feeding: Third Report. Report on Health and Social Subjects No. 32. Her Majesty's Stationery Office, London
4. Hamilton E M N, Whitney E N 1979 Nutrition: Concepts and Controversies. West Publishing Co., St. Paul, Minnesota
5. Truswell A S 1985 ABC of Nutrition: Children and Adolescents. British Medical Journal 291: 397
6. Benton D, Roberts G 1988 Effect of Vitamin and Mineral Supplementation on Intelligence of a Sample of Schoolchildren. Lancet 8578: 140
7. Bull N L 1988 Studies of Dietary Habits, Food Consumption and Nutrient Intake of Adolescents and Young Adults. World Review of Nutrition and Dietetics 57: 24
8. Smith N J 1983 Physical Activity and Dietary Intakes. In: White P L, Mondeika T (eds) Diet and exercise: Synergism in Health Maintenance. American Medical Association, Chicago, p 27
9. Nutrition Committee, Canadian Paediatric Society 1983 Adolescent Nutrition: 4. Sports and Diet. Canadian Medical Association Journal 129: 552
10. Rowland T W 1989 Medical Concerns for Child Athletes. Sports Medicine Digest 11 (3): 1
11. Department of Health and Social Security, Committee on Medical Aspects of Food Policy 1989 The Diets of British Schoolchildren. Report on Health and Social Subjects No. 36. Her Majesty's Stationery Office, London
12. Mahlamaki E, Mahlamaki S 1988 Iron Deficiency in Adolescent Female Dancers. British Journal of Sports Medicine 22 (2): 55–56
13. Mirkin G 1987 Eating for Competition. Seminars in Adolescent Medicine 3 (3): 177

Suggested further reading
GENERAL NUTRITION
The Everyman Companion to Food and Nutrition. Sheila Bingham. 1987. J M Dent.
The Family Guide to Food and Health. Elisabeth Morse, John Rivers and Anne Heughan. 1988. Barrie and Jenkins.
The Penguin Encyclopaedia of Nutrition. John Yudkin. 1985. Penguin Books.

CHILDREN'S NUTRITION

Healthy Eating for Your Child. Heather Bampfylde and John Dickerson. 1985. William Collins.

Eat It Up – A parent's guide to eating problems. Dr David Haslam. 1986. Macdonald.

Nutrition for Children. D Francis. 1987. Blackwell Scientific Publications.

Cooking for Kids the Healthy Way. Joanna Pay. 1986. Martin Dunitz.

Handbook of Child Nutrition. L S Taitz and B Wardley. 1989. Oxford Medical Publications.

SPORTS NUTRITION

Food for Action. 1987. Pelham Books.

Food for Sport. Karen Inge and Peter Bruckner. 1988. The Kingswood Press.

Eating for Peak Performance. Rosemary Stanton. 1988. Unwin Hyman.

Nutrition for Sport. Steve Wootton. 1988. Simon & Schuster.

Too Thin to Win. An information booklet on eating disorders. Produced under the auspices of the International Athletic Foundation. 1989. Available from IAAF, 3 Hans Crescent, London SW1.

Index

Abdomen, 37, 146
Abdominal muscles, 140, 144, 146, 147; pains, 72, 183
Accessory movements, 62
Accident(s), 81, 93
Achilles (calcaneal) tendon(s), 61, 91, 126, 134, 138
Acrocyanosis, 195
Acromioclavicular joint, 148
Additives, 183
Adductor muscles, 143
Adipose tissue, 37
Adolescence, 1, 39, 188
Adolescent(s), 33, 38, 39, 40, 44, 45, 55, 69, 71, 133, 194, 201, 203, 205, 207
Adult fitness equations, 61
Aerobic capacity, 33; energy, 44; events, 66; fitness, 47–8; fitness tests, 54–7; power, 54, 59, 70; performance, 51; training, 27, 53
Aerobics, 173
Age, 36, 54
Age groups, 1, 21, 36, 76
Age limits, 15
Aggression, 3
Air pollutants, 51
Alcohol, 190
Allergies, 72
Allergy clinic, 184
Altitude training, 59
Amateur Athletics Association, 15, 20
Amateur Rowing Association, 18
Amateur sport, 7
Amateur Swimming Association, 15, 20

Ambition, 10
Amenorrhoea, 37, 39, 40, 123, 195, 205
American Academy of Pediatrics, 43
American College of Sports Medicine, 32
American football, 36, 85, 89, 129, 137, 146, 148, 151, 156
Ampler, Uwe, 8
Anabolic effect, 43
Anabolic steroids, 35
Anaemia, 194, 200
Anaerobic activity, 66; capacity, 33, 34; endurance, 71; energy, 44; fitness, 44–7; power, 44; tests, 44–7; threshold, 44, 57; training, 28
Ankle(s), 63, 72, 134, 136–8, 152, 165
Anorexia nervosa, 39, 195–6
Anterior tibial muscles, 139
Anti-gravity muscles, 145
Anti-tetanus injections, 81
Antibiotics, 93, 120
Apophyseal avulsion fracture, 130
Apophysis, 126–30
Apophysitis, 116, 127
Appetite, 179, 186
Arm(s), 34, 37, 64, 73, 79, 84, 87, 112, 129
Arm-bone (humerus), 34, 62, 124, 149, 150
Arthritis, 135
Arthroscopy, 154, 159
Artificial colours (in food), 183
Artificial flavours (in food), 183
Artificial respiration, 79

Artificial surfaces, 153
Aspirin, 72
Assisted passive stretching, 65
Asthma, 4, 50, 60, 80, 183
Atherosclerosis, 40, 48, 54, 60
Athletic trainer, 98
Athletics, 17, 19, 205
Australia, 8, 194
Avulsion fracture, 117

Babies, 1, 5, 22–3, 96, 138, 165, 175
Back (trunk), 24, 34, 39, 64, 76, 85, 93, 120, 137, 140, 141, 143, 147, 152, 169, 172, 173
Backbone (vertebral column), 33, 36, 195
Badminton, 91, 138, 147, 166, 169
Balance, 70, 135, 136, 137, 139, 144, 151, 165, 172; tests, 100
Ball skills, 22, 82, 151
Ballet, 201
Ballistic exercises, 64
Bandaging, 80, 129, 139, 153
Bar-Or, Oded, 45
Basal pulse, 99
Baseball, 148, 149
Basic Four Food Groups, 177, 186
Basketball, 137, 138, 151
Bath, 65, 90, 170
Bed-rest, 49, 93, 130
Bell-ringing, 211
Bi-acromial breadth, 34
Bicycle(s), 23, 85
Biological age, 36
Biological ratio standards, 54
Biomechanical inefficiency, 60, 68; monitoring, 27, 96–114
Bipartite patella, 122
Bisham Abbey National Sports Centre, 8
Bleeding, 80, 120
Blister(s), 91
Blood, 33, 40, 48, 54, 80, 153, 177; fats, 39–41; gas analysis, 57; lactate levels, 69; lactic acid, 46, 57; lipid profiles, 40; pressure, 48,

52, 53, 175; tests, 152, 173, 174; vessels, 155
Body mass index, 195
Body proportions, 33, 66, 133
Body surface to weight ratio, 67
Body water, 50
Bodyweight, 36, 37, 45, 51, 54, 59, 67, 68, 158, 195, 202, 210
Bone(s), 40, 41, 62, 94, 132, 177; cyst, 74; density, 189; development, 33; diseases, 130–1; fractures, 40, 79, 116–26; fusion, 35, 116, 133; graft, 75; growth, 1, 33–5, 43, 116, 155; injuries, 34–5, 44, 79, 116–31; scan, 125, 170
Boys' Brigade, 211
Box(es) (for genital protection), 85
Boxing, 14, 85, 89, 208
Brace, 125, 155
Brachialis, 150
Brain, 41, 79, 120
Breast-bone (sternum), 107, 148
Breathing, 49–52; exercises, 50; rates, 49, 69
Britain, 8, 10, 97, 175, 185, 195
British Amateur Gymnastics Association, 16
Bronchi, 47, 51
Bronchial cancer, 50
Brown fat, 39
Brownies, 211
Bruise, bruising, 79, 118, 120
Bulimia nervosa, 195–6
'Bullworker', 110
Bunion(s), 90, 134–5
'Burn-out', 211
Bursa(e), 132
Bursitis, 144
Buxton, Angela, 9

Calcaneal apophysitis, 128
Calcaneal (Achilles) tendon, 61, 91, 126, 134, 138
Calcium, 40, 177, 188, 194, 203
Calf muscles, 42, 45, 72, 101, 138, 141, 152, 156, 160, 165, 168

Callipers, 37
Calories, 38, 40, 176, 197, 203
Canoeing, 34, 44, 53, 87;
    ergometer, 33
Capillary function, 48, 49
Capsule, 62, 132, 137
Carbohydrate(s), 197, 202, 203, 206,
    208
Carbohydrate loading, 205
Carbohydrate polymers, 208
Carbon dioxide, 33, 48, 50
Cardiac arrhythmias, 205;
    development, 53; dilatation, 53;
    hypertrophy, 52; massage, 79;
    output, 68; threshold, 57
Cardiorespiratory-haemic axis, 58
Cardiorespiratory system, 57
Cardiovascular system, 68
'Carrying angle', 35
Carter, Cyril, Rita, Sharon,
    Christina, 18–21
Cartilage, 116, 119, 144, 154, 159
Cartilages (menisci), 132, 153, 156
Casualty officer, doctor, 153
Centre of ossification, 116
Cereals, 177, 181, 183, 186, 190,
    198, 200, 207, 208
'Charley-horse' injury, 141
Chartered physiotherapist, 27, 64,
    91, 96, 97, 98, 99, 114, 125, 129,
    135, 138, 142, 147, 151, 160, 171
Chemical fats, 37
Chest, 34, 110, 144, 147
Chewing gum, 81
Child abuse, 71
Chiropodist (podiatrist), 91, 136,
    138, 161
Chiropractor, 147
Cholesterol, 37
Chondromalacia patellae, 159
Chronic bronchitis, 50
Chronological age, 36
'Cinema sign', 158
Circuit training, 27–8, 30
Circulation, 68, 80, 125, 131
Clarke's sign, 160

Clavicle (collar-bone), 148
Clay pigeon shooting, 85
'Clicking' joints, 72, 118, 119
Climbing, 40
Climbing frame, 2, 22
Clothing, 89, 90, 100, 114
Coach(es), 6, 7, 8, 9, 17, 18, 27, 36,
    41, 44, 64, 70, 76, 81, 84, 86, 89,
    98, 99, 114, 150, 170, 172, 204,
    211
Cognitive function, 200
Cold conditions, environment, 30,
    40, 50, 60, 68, 90, 201
Collar-bone (clavicle), 148
Committee on Medical Aspects of
    Food Policy (COMA), 179
Compartment syndrome, 139
Competition(s), 10, 23, 29, 32, 35,
    82, 124, 196, 205, 206, 211
Competitive sport, 4, 8, 11, 12–15,
    16, 23, 58, 70, 98, 115, 169, 170
Competitors, 26, 35, 44, 53, 66, 68,
    97
Concentration, 3, 8
Concentric muscle work, 25, 29
Concussion, 119
Conditioning, 21, 30
Confidence, 22, 210
Constipation, 196
'Contagious hysteria', 50
Contraceptive pill, 40
Convection, 67
Cooper 12-minute run test
    equation, 61
Co-ordination, 1, 70, 92, 99, 102,
    113, 136, 137, 139, 142, 149,
    151, 159, 161, 166, 182, 210
Coronary artery disease, 40
Corset, 147, 174
Council of Europe, 96
Cramp(s), 90, 123, 138, 207
Creatine-phosphate, 45
Cricket, 13, 85, 151, 164, 212
Crutches, 80, 125, 139
Crystal Palace National Sports
    Centre Injuries Unit, 75

Cubs, 211
Cybex (muscle measuring apparatus), 95, 141, 142
Cycle ergometer, 33, 45, 57
Cycle tests, 55
Cycling, 23, 26, 27, 52, 61, 66, 85, 88, 125, 159, 167, 182
Czechoslovakia, 8

Dance, 32, 40, 173, 210
Dancers, 63
David exercise system, 29, 144
Death, 48–9, 74
Decathlon, 25
Dedication, 3
Degenerative joint disease (osteoarthritis), 78, 98, 119, 152
Dehydration, 33, 47, 68, 69, 70, 90, 201, 204, 207
Dental care, 98
Dentist(s), 85
Department of Health and Social Security, 179
Determination, 3, 8, 78
Diabetes, 80
Diagnosis, 73, 124, 143, 153, 154, 160, 171, 182, 184
Diaphysis, 116
Diarrhoea, 207
Diastolic pressure, 48, 52
Diet(s), 41, 59, 98, 126, 133, 152, 174, 175–209, 210
Dietary deficiencies, 123, 133, 196
Dietary manipulation, 39, 183
Dietary supplements, 193
Dietician(s), 126, 184, 194, 195
Disappointment, 82
Discipline, 89
Discoid meniscus, 154
Discs, 132, 147
Disease, 135, 175
Disorientation, 68
Diuretics, 195, 204
Divers, 123
Diving, 28, 31, 42
Doctor(s), 40, 50, 73, 74, 75, 79, 81, 98, 100, 114, 115, 124, 127, 129, 130, 136, 143, 152, 165, 166, 175, 182, 194
Dressings, 79
Drink(s), 68, 69, 180, 198, 201
Drugs, 35, 37
Dynamic exercise(s), 30, 52
Dynamometer, 42, 114

Ears, 120
Ear defenders, 85
East Germany, 8
Eccentric muscle work, 25, 29, 162
Education Act, 185
Edwards, Eddie 'The Eagle', 7
Elastic strain energy, 61
Elbow(s), 35, 62, 79, 85, 112, 124, 149–51, 170
Electrical muscle stimulation, 122, 125, 129, 136, 138, 139, 149, 155, 160–1, 166, 167, 168, 169, 171, 172
Electrocardiograph changes, 53
Electrolyte imbalances, 205
Electrolyte replacement drink, 69
Electrotherapy, 129, 155
Elite sport, 7, 32, 39, 44, 55, 59, 60, 63, 65, 71, 75, 76, 97
Emergency treatments, 79, 139, 143, 155
Endurance, 57, 58, 66, 68, 69, 70
Energy, 37, 47, 50, 54, 66, 175, 176, 188, 197, 200, 202, 203
Energy storage capacity, 61
England boys' squash squads, 56, 76–8, 97
Epiphyseal plates, 33, 35, 116
Epiphysis, 90, 116, 127, 129
Epiphysitis, 127
Equipment, 84–6, 114, 150, 170
Ergometers, 33
Erzberger, Peter, 13
Euphoria, 68
Excitability, 68
Exercise physiology, 32–71; testing, 57; therapy, 133

Exercise-induced asthma, 50
Exhaustion, 70
Eye–hand co-ordination, 22, 82

Face, 122; -mask, 85
Failure, 6, 8, 36
Families, 5, 10–21, 166, 210
Family doctor (general practitioner), 74, 100, 152, 164
Fast foods, 193
Fast muscle, 66
Fat, 37–41, 48, 68, 132, 175, 179, 197, 200, 203, 204; pads, 132, 156; percentage(s), 37, 54, 194
Fatigue, 1, 26, 42, 44, 46, 60, 70, 83, 87, 92, 99, 138, 197, 211
Fear, 22
Feingold, Ben, 183
Fell walking, 66
Femoral version, 140
Femur (thigh-bone), 34, 74, 118, 124, 125, 129, 130, 140, 152, 156, 159
Fencing, 85, 159
Fever, 49
Fibre, 177, 179
Fibula, 34, 124, 125, 152
Field tests, 54–6
Finger(s), 73, 113, 151
First-aid, 79–81
Fish, 178, 184, 186, 190, 194, 199, 200, 203
Fisk, John, 14
Fitness, 47, 58, 97, 213; programmes, 3, 30; training, 24, 26–31, 87, 115, 211
Flat feet, 82, 91, 134, 135, 156, 165
Flexibility, 22, 29, 61–6, 95, 99, 138; tests, 29, 64; training, 29, 156
Fluid, 138, 201–4
Food intolerance, 183–4
Foot, 33, 61, 63, 72, 82, 90, 125, 130, 133, 134–6, 140, 152, 156, 166
Football (soccer), 2, 8, 24, 32, 47, 52, 76, 82, 86, 89, 97, 129, 138, 143, 146, 153, 155, 157, 201
Forearm, 34, 63, 112, 150
Fracture(s), 79, 117–26, 146, 151, 154
Free fatty acids, 37
Freiburg's disease, 130
Friction characteristics of shoes, 91
Friedrich, Heike, 8
Friendships, 8, 16, 210
Fruit(s), 177, 180, 181, 183, 186, 198, 200

'Gamekeeper's thumb', 151
Gastrointestinal function, 200; problems, 205
General practitioner (family doctor), 74, 100, 152, 164
Genetic factors, 61
Genu recurvatum, 156
Girl Guides, 211
'Giving way' (of joint), 119, 154
Glandular fever, 49
Glucose, 44, 48
Glycogen, 44, 60, 197, 205
Goggles, 85
Golf, 13, 20, 28, 86, 212
'Golfer's elbow', 171
Goniometer, 64
Governing body, 7
Governments, 3
Gravity, 25; centre of, 34, 40
Greenstick fracture(s), 117
Grip strength, 35, 41, 114
Groin, 118, 143
'Growing pains', 72, 138, 166
Growth, 3, 35, 39, 42, 57, 98, 132, 156, 158, 166, 167, 192, 204, 210
Growth plate (physis), 35, 116, 120, 133, 137, 143, 146, 149
Growth spurt, 14, 30, 33, 34, 35, 36, 37, 42, 54, 59, 60, 63, 82, 94, 132, 140, 141, 157, 188
Gum shields, 85
'Gym-Joey', 70
Gymnastics, 6, 10, 14, 16–17, 19, 23, 26, 29, 30, 32, 34, 40, 44, 53, 63,

82, 97, 120, 135, 137, 138, 146, 148, 149, 150, 170, 208, 211
Gymnasts, 37, 41, 63, 123, 124, 169, 172

Haemoglobin, 48, 51, 59
Hamstrings, 64, 104, 141, 155, 157, 160, 168, 173
Hand(s), 33, 151, 171
'Hard tissues', 132
Hay fever, 183
Head injury, 119
Headaches, 78, 183
Health education programmes, 3, 175; screening, 96, 98
Health-promoting exercise, 3, 32
Heart, 33, 48, 58; disease, 6, 48, 175; growth, 58; malformation, 48; rate(s), 33, 48, 52, 53, 57, 59; volume, 53
Heat, 39, 66, 80; control, 33, 66; gradient, 67; lamp, 80
Heel(s), 34, 90, 126, 128, 134
Heel tabs, 91, 138
Height, 33, 54, 99, 116, 194
Hellmann, Martina, 9
Helmet, 85
Heredity, 132, 135, 156
Hernia, 143
Heterotopic ossification, 150
High jump, 35, 120
High-density lipoproteins (HDL), 40
Hip(s), 34, 37, 62, 72, 76, 78, 84, 90, 105, 106, 108, 110, 118, 127, 130, 143–4, 152, 164, 168, 170, 172, 174, 195
Hip abductor muscles, 107
Hockey, 24, 47, 51, 52, 85, 91, 123, 148, 158, 165
Hormones, 43
Hospital, 74, 79, 81, 96, 118, 120, 125, 149, 155, 163, 169, 173
Hot weather conditions, 67–8
Hoyt, Gary, 14
Human foetus, 59
Humerus (arm-bone), 34, 62, 124, 149, 150
Hurdling, 129
Hydrafitness exercise system, 29
Hydraulic resistance equipment, 28, 29
Hyperactive Children's Support Group, 183, 209
Hyperactivity, 182, 195
Hypermobility, 63
Hypertrophy, 41, 43, 53
Hyperventilation hypocapnia, 50
Hypoactive children, 41
Hypothermia, 68, 90

Ice hockey, 85, 148, 158
Ice treatment, 79, 80, 125, 129, 139, 153, 157, 172
Ice-skaters, 52
Ice-skating, 10, 40
Idiopathic kyphosis, 131
Idiopathic scoliosis, 131
Iliac crest, 128
Ilium, 143
Illness, 27, 60, 92, 115, 125, 126, 211
Immunological system, 184, 200
India, 8
Individual sports, 2, 7, 23, 89
Individuality, 3, 26
Infants, 38, 51
Infection, 60, 69, 79, 81, 85, 93, 99, 100, 124
Inflammatory arthritis, 152, 174
Inhibition, 133
Institute of Child Health, 97
Interferential therapy, 149
International Olympic Committee, 7
Interval training, 28
Intrinsic muscles, 135
Iron, 177, 190–2, 200, 203
Ischaemia, 139
Isometric muscle work, 53
Isotonic drinks, 208
Isotonic exercise, 52

Jacuzzi, 81

Javelin throwing, 42, 79, 88, 149, 150
Jewellery, 89
Jogging, 197
Joint(s), 26, 29, 33, 61, 62, 64, 72, 132, 149, 154
Judo, 89, 146, 148
Jumping, 28, 43, 51, 66, 82, 91, 129, 134, 135, 157, 165
'Junk food', 39

Karate, 28, 129, 155, 166, 167, 212
Kin-Com (muscle measuring apparatus), 95, 141, 142
Kicking (a ball), 134, 164
Kinetic balance, 61
'Kiss of life', 79
Knee(s), 62, 72, 76, 78, 84, 85, 90, 103, 119, 134, 137, 140, 141, 143, 152–63, 164, 166, 167; cartilage(s), 153–4; cruciate ligaments, 154–5; dislocation, 155; fat pad impingement, 156; medial ligament, 155; plica, 157
Knee-cap (patellofemoral) joint, 85, 140; chondromalacia, 159; dislocation, 163, 169; pain syndrome, 76, 140, 158–63; subluxation, 140, 163
Knock-knees, 140
Kohler's disease, 130
Korbut, Olga, 6
Kyphosis, 131

Laboratory tests, 41, 45, 52, 54, 70, 97, 98
Lacrosse, 51, 52
Lactate threshold, 57
Lactic acid, 28, 33, 44, 57
Laser therapy, 149
Lateral femoral torsion, 140
Lateral release operation, 162, 167
Lawn Tennis Association, 9
Laxatives, 195, 204
Leg(s), 33, 34, 64, 72, 78, 87, 90, 94, 100, 122, 133, 134–9
Leg length discrepancy, 146

Legg-Calvé-Perthes disease, 131
Lendl, Ivan, 8
Lessmann, Erika, 14
Levers, 41, 84, 139
Lido (muscle measuring apparatus), 95, 141, 142
Life-saving, 79
Lifting, 146, 173
Ligament(s), 62, 73, 132, 144, 150, 151, 154
Lilleshall National Sports Centre, 8
Limitation of joint movement, 61
Limp, 75, 118, 122, 123, 126, 129, 138, 139, 154, 159, 165
Litigation, 97
Little Athletic Clubs, 66
'Little League Elbow', 149
Liver glycogen, 197, 207
Local muscle endurance, 33, 44
'Locking', 119, 171
Long plantar ligament, 135
Loose bodies, 119, 154
Lordosis, 63, 140, 146, 170
Lumbar spine, 63, 107, 154
Lung(s), 33, 47, 49, 51, 54

Macdonald-Smith, Iain, 13
MacDougal equation, 61
McIntyre, Mike, 12–15; Caroline, Angus, Gemma, 14–15
Magaria step-running test, 45
Malignant tumour, 74
Malnutrition, 35, 204
Manager, 211
Manipulation, 73, 147, 172
Maradonna, Diego, 8
Marathon running, 15, 17, 32, 36, 60, 66, 205
Marker, 89
Massage, 141, 147, 157
Matron, 169
Maturation, 54
Maturity, 66, 71, 89, 94, 116, 212
Maximum heart rates, 52
Meat(s), 178, 181, 186, 200, 206
Medial femoral torsion, 140

Medical advice, 37, 40
Medical officer, 80, 96, 115
Medical problems, 4, 98
Medical specialists, 6, 15
Medical treatment, 80, 149
Menarche, 37
Meniscectomy, 154
Menisci (cartilages), 132, 153, 156
Menstruation (periods), 36, 39, 201
Metabolic function, 57
Metabolic specialists, 66
Metabolism, 33, 45, 66, 69
Metacarpophalangeal joints, 151
Metaphysis, 116
Metatarsal bone, 125, 130
Milk, 40, 176, 180, 203
Millfield School, 20
Minerals, 133, 176, 188, 193, 197
Mini-rugby, 70, 82, 114
Mitochondria, 48, 49
Mixed competitions, 35
Mobility, 29, 33, 61–6
Mobilizations, 172, 173
Mobilizing exercises, 29, 30, 64, 99,
    150, 164
Monitoring, 20, 27, 44, 64, 76, 96,
    114, 115, 120, 134, 167
Moser, Constanze, 9
Motivation, 10, 45, 58, 60, 70, 76
Motor nerves, 41
Motor rallying, 12
Motorbike scrambling, 120, 146
Mountain walking, 66
Movement, 1
Movement economy, 33, 60–1
Multistage 20-metre shuttle run
    test, 55
Muscle, 1, 29, 33, 41, 58, 60, 62, 66,
    71, 82, 94, 129, 132, 140; cell(s),
    44, 48; contraction speed, 42;
    elasticity, 62, 64, 87; endurance,
    28, 33, 87, 109, 110; enzymes, 60;
    fascia, 139; fatigue, 62, 97; fibre
    profile, 66; hypertrophy, 41;
    imbalance, 139, 141, 149, 173;
    power, 41; protein synthesis, 41;
spasm, 123, 140, 143; speed, 33;
    strength, 29, 33, 41, 64; tightness,
    29, 30, 62, 65; tone, 125, 145,
    210; versatility, 33, 66; weakness,
    62
'Muscle-bound', 29, 95
Muscle–tendon unit, 132
Musculoskeletal problems, 75
Musculoskeletal system, 41
Myogenic component of strength, 41
Myoglobin, 48, 49
Myositis ossificans, 80, 141

Nautilus exercise system, 29, 144
Navratilova, Martina, 8
Neck, 110, 144, 148, 173, 174
Nerve(s), 37, 137, 141, 155, 171
Nerve conduction tests, 171
Nervous system, 41
Netball, 129, 138, 166
Neurogenic aspect of
    strength gain, 41
Neuromuscular development, 71
Norman, Ross, 7
Norsk exercise system, 27, 28, 29,
    144, 147, 172, 173
Nose, 120
Nurse, 96
Nutrients, 175
Nutritional advice, 37
Nutritional supplements, 205
Nutritionist, 126, 175

Obesity, 26, 38, 68, 175, 182, 187,
    194
Occupational therapist, 91
Oedema, 196
Oesophageal tears, 205
Oestrogen, 40
Oligomenorrhoea, 205
Olympic Games, 6, 7, 12, 15, 19
Onset of blood lactate accumulation
    (OBLA), 57
Organ(s), 37, 132, 147
Orthopaedic specialist, surgeon, 73,
    74, 118, 153, 154, 155, 159, 167,
    171

Orthotics, 91, 136, 138, 161
Osgood-Schlatter's 'disease', 76, 128, 157
Ossification, 36, 116, 149
Osteoarthritis (degenerative joint disease), 78, 98, 119, 156
Osteochondral fracture, 119
Osteochondritis, 130; dissecans, 119, 156
Osteomyelitis, 120, 124
Osteopath, 147, 167, 172
Osteoporosis, 40, 189, 205
Otto, Kristin, 8
Overcooling, 68
Overeating, 38
Over-exercising, 39, 83, 143, 147
Over-heating, 47, 67, 70
Over-pronation, 135, 139
Over-specialization, 24, 66, 114, 211
Over-stretching, 64, 65, 139, 141, 147
Over-supination, 135
Over-training, 79, 83, 87, 98, 126
Overuse injuries, 64, 87, 117, 127, 133, 141, 150, 151, 152, 157, 159, 171
Oxidative enzymes, 58
Oxygen consumption, 33; cost, 60; debt, 45–6; deficit, 69; uptake, 39, 54–5, 69

Paediatric specialist(s), 118, 122, 131
Page, Cheryl, Pamela, Brian, Dorothy, 15–18
Pain, 44, 72, 92, 115, 118, 123, 126, 129, 135, 136, 139, 140, 144, 147, 153, 165, 167, 169, 170, 172
Paralysis, 120
Parent(s), 3, 4, 6, 7, 9, 27, 51, 73, 76, 80, 84, 92, 99, 129, 135, 160, 167, 175, 182, 195, 210, 211
Pars interarticularis, 123
Passive range of movement, 62
Passive smoking, 51
Passive stretching exercises, 29, 64, 138, 141

Patella (knee-cap), 152, 168; alta, 156
Patellar tendon, 127, 140, 152, 157, 166, 168
Patellofemoral (knee-cap) joint, 152
Pattinson, Rodney, 13
Peak height velocity, 188
Pelvis, 34, 106, 109, 124, 130, 134, 137, 140, 141, 143, 146, 170
Pentathlon, 25
Percentage fat, 33
Periods (menstruation), 36, 39, 40
Perthes' disease, 131
Physical education, 3, 4, 56, 75, 213
Physical educationist(s), 3, 5, 36, 89, 96
Physical fitness, 2, 22, 32
Physiological monitoring, 20, 27, 57, 96
Physiologist(s), 27, 62, 64, 97, 98
Physiotherapist(s) (Chartered), 27, 64, 91, 96, 97, 98, 99, 114, 125, 129, 135, 138, 142, 147, 151, 160, 171
Physiotherapy, 139, 144, 149, 154, 155, 157, 158, 162, 163, 164, 165, 167, 169, 171, 173
Physis (growth plate), 35, 116, 121, 133, 137, 143, 146, 149
'Pigeon-toes', 140
Plantar fascia, 135
Plaster cast, 119, 125, 129, 151, 167, 169
Play, 1, 75
Pleasure, 1, 3
Podiatrist, 91, 136, 138, 161
'Ponderostat', 39
Post-exercise oxygen consumption test, 45
Post-pubescent(s), post-pubertal, 1, 52, 204
Posture, 5, 25–6, 30, 98, 131, 144–5, 147, 156, 172, 210, 211
Potassium chloride, 69
Power, 41
Power training, 28

Powerlifting, 29, 43, 94
Pre-adolescent(s), 43, 47
Pre-participation assessment, 97
Pre-pubescent(s), pre-pubertal, 1, 37, 40, 43, 54, 59, 201
Pre-school children, 178
Pre-teen, 1, 60, 64, 74, 82, 120
Pregnancy, 200
Pressure, 9, 10, 11, 211
Professional sport, 6, 11, 172, 211
'Programme for life', 19–21
Proprioception, 137
Protective equipment, 85, 115
Protective exercises, 25, 30–1, 87, 172, 174, 211
Protein, 176, 188, 197, 199
Psychiatrist, 195
Psychological problems, 24, 205
Psychomotor system, 41
Puberty, 1, 34, 36, 40, 42, 43, 52, 53, 59, 66, 67, 70, 132, 140
Publicity, 20
Pulmonary ventilation, 57
Pulse rate, 48, 99, 100, 184
'Pump bump', 91

Quadriceps muscles, 45, 74, 103, 140, 141, 156, 160, 175
'Q-angle', 156

Racket sports, 26, 34, 82, 129, 149
Racketball, 70
Radiation, 67
Radius, 34, 150
'Reasonable exercise', 79
Rebound movement, 61
Recommended Daily Amounts (RDA) of food energy, 179, 197, 201
Recovery, 26, 30, 69, 92, 126, 150, 162, 208
Rectus femoris muscle, 140
Referee, 2, 89
Referred pain, 120, 141, 143, 146
Rehabilitation, 92, 122, 147, 150, 154, 155

Relationships, 6, 7, 8, 9, 98
Relaxation, 5, 26
Remedial exercises, 31, 43, 78, 99, 115, 119, 125, 131, 136, 137, 138, 141, 142, 144, 149, 151, 154, 155, 158, 161, 168, 169, 172, 173
Repetitive training, 27, 35, 83, 123
Resistance training, 29, 42–3
Respiratory rate, 49
Rest, 26, 28, 30, 47, 60, 68, 93, 125, 126, 130
Resuscitation, 80
Retropatellar pain, 158–63
Rewards, 3, 6, 7, 14
Rheumatic fever, 49
Rheumatologist, 152, 166, 170, 171, 173
Rib(s), 93, 124
Riding, 13, 20, 82, 85, 146, 149
Roller skating, 2, 4, 153
Rounders, 166
Rowers, 26, 145
Rowing, 24, 34, 44, 53, 74, 83, 87, 123, 145, 212; ergometer, 33
Royal Life Saving Society, 20
Rugby, 13, 32, 36, 42, 51, 82, 89, 120, 129, 146, 148
Rules, 2, 89, 114
'Runner's knee', 158–63
Runners, 55, 83, 91, 124, 207
Running, 22, 24, 27, 32, 44, 47, 51, 52, 53, 60, 61, 65, 76, 79, 83, 87, 123, 124, 129, 134, 135, 141, 143, 157, 159, 165, 197, 212
Running economy, 60

Sailing, 12, 40
Salicylates, 183
Salt (Sodium chloride), 69, 175, 180
Salt tablets, 202
Sartorius muscle, 140
Scapula (shoulder blade), 93, 148, 174, 195
Scheuermann's disease, 131
Schnell exercise system, 29

School, 3, 6, 20, 80, 89, 96, 98, 115, 166, 169, 184, 212
'School of Sport', 165
School Sport Forum, 32
Scoliosis, 145
Scouts, 211
Second wind, 46
Secondary injuries, 133, 140, 151, 152, 157, 159
Seles, Monica, 8
Self-esteem, 3, 131, 210
Sever's 'disease', 127, 128
Sex, 36, 54
Sexual development, 36, 192
Sexual interference, 9
Shin guard(s), 85
Shin soreness, 83
Shin-bone (tibia), 124, 125, 140, 156
Shinty, 51
Shivering, 67
Shoes, 90, 99, 100, 133, 135, 137, 139, 156, 165
Short tennis, 20, 23, 70, 82, 114
Shot-putting, 42
Shoulder(s), 34, 62, 83, 87, 111, 127, 129, 146, 148–50, 172; blade (scapula), 93, 148, 174, 195; dislocation, 149; subluxation, 149
Shoulder girdle, 93
Shower, 65, 90
Sinding-Larsen-Johannson 'disease', 128, 157
Sit-and-reach test, 64
Sitting height, 34
Six-minute endurance run test, 56
Size, 66, 82; -matching, 89, 146
Skateboarding, 2, 85, 151, 153
Skiing, 23, 89, 124, 149, 151, 155, 159, 166, 167; ergometer, 33
Skill(s), 1, 8, 15, 21, 22, 30, 44, 66, 70, 86, 114, 210
Skin, 67, 68, 79, 100, 120, 137, 196, 201
Skinfold measurements, 37, 38
Skipping, 27, 53, 124
Skull, 85, 120

Skylarking, 76
Sling, 80, 149, 171
Slipped capital femoral epiphysis, 118
Smoking, 50–2, 60, 175, 190
'Snapping hips', 144
Soccer (football), 51, 164, 166
Sodium chloride (salt), 69, 175, 180
Soft-ball cricket, 70
'Soft-tissues', 29, 132–51, 210
Somatotype, 54, 66
Soviet Union, 8
Specialization, 6, 8, 21, 23, 25, 66
Speed training, 28, 30
Speed-power, 41
Sphygmomanometer, 48
Spinal cord, 41, 120
Spine, 24, 26, 28, 79, 123, 124, 131, 145
Spleen, 147
Splints, 79, 119
Splits, 143, 155
Spondylolisthesis, 124, 125
Spondylolysis, 123, 124
Sponsorship, 20
Sport: as a career, 4, 6, 24, 172, 211; as entertainment, 4; as specialized competition, 4, 6; beneficial effects of, 4, 5; competitive, 4; definition of, 1; National Institute(s) of, 8
Sports: acrobatics, 172; centre(s), 3, 7, 9, 80, 98, 212; clinic, 75; clubs, 7, 9, 80, 85, 98, 212; halls, 69, 89; physiologist, 27; psychologist, 11; star, 3, 8, 15
Sportsmanship, 3
Sprain(s), 79, 133
Sprinting, 28, 44, 51, 66, 141
Squads, 7, 11, 14, 56, 69, 70, 75, 76, 97, 124
Squash, 11, 14, 32, 47, 51, 56, 61, 63, 69, 76–8, 83, 87, 89, 91, 124, 129, 138, 147, 155, 157, 158
Squat-and-reach endurance test, 105
Stability, 30, 34

Stabilometer, 34
Staleness, 98
Stamina, 57, 60
Starvation, 204
Static muscle work, 53
Static stretching, 64
Step-Test, 56
Sternoclavicular joint, 148
Sternum (breast-bone), 107, 148
Steward, Len, 11
'Stitch', 146
Stratton, Vernon, 14
Strength, 22, 28, 29, 35, 41, 42–4,
    70, 87, 92, 99, 130, 131
Strength-power, 41
Strengthening exercises, 166, 170
Stress, 24, 29; fractures, 40, 87, 117,
    122–6, 205
Stretcher, 80
Stretching exercises, 29, 30, 87, 99,
    130, 131, 138, 164, 171
Stroke volume, 48, 53
Sudden death, 48–9
Sugar, 69, 175, 180, 206
'Superstars', 18
Supervision, 29, 88, 114
Suppling, 21
Surfing, 89
Surgery, 125, 130, 139, 141, 144,
    147, 151, 153, 155, 157, 158,
    162, 163
Survival skills, 3
Sweating, 67, 69, 90, 201
Swelling, 80, 90, 92, 118, 123, 151,
    152, 153, 155
'Swim-bench', 28
Swimmer(s), 41, 43, 65, 68, 149,
    168, 207
'Swimmer's shoulder', 149
Swimming, 5, 10, 12, 13, 15, 16, 19,
    22, 24, 27, 32, 37, 40, 44, 51, 52,
    53, 83, 97, 125, 144, 147, 155,
    164, 165, 167, 182, 208
Swimming pool(s), 80
Synovial fluid, 62, 132, 153
Synthetic surfaces, 83

Systolic pressure, 48, 52

Tactical skills, 3
Tae Kwon Do, 85
Talent, 4, 8, 23, 82, 97, 98, 210
Taping, 137, 151
Teacher(s), 3, 4, 5, 76, 81, 86, 89,
    96, 114, 129, 165
Team(s), 2, 69, 89, 165
Teamwork, 3
Technique, 86, 114, 150, 211
Teen(s), 3, 74, 133, 136, 140
Teenagers, 1, 6, 9, 25, 26, 27, 29, 30,
    39, 40, 64, 78, 79, 87, 88, 95, 99,
    124, 133, 138, 140, 141, 143,
    144, 148, 153, 158, 159, 160,
    187–94, 210
Teeth, 205
Television, 3, 5, 20, 26, 89, 145, 159,
    210
Temperature, 49, 66–8, 69, 89, 99,
    201
Temple, Cliff, 20
Tendon(s), 41, 61, 83, 116, 126, 127,
    130, 132, 137, 144, 150, 151
Tennis, 8, 9, 13, 19, 24, 28, 35, 44,
    82, 84, 86, 91, 97, 124, 143, 145,
    149, 164, 165, 166, 170, 211, 212
'Tennis elbow', 150
Tennis players, 43, 149
The Sports Council, 97
Thermometer, 99
Thermoregulation, 204
Thigh, 37, 74, 83, 140–4, 152, 168
Thigh-bone (femur), 34, 74, 118,
    124, 125, 129, 130, 140, 152,
    156, 159
Thirst, 69, 207
'Thirst fever', 69
Thoracic spine (mid-back), 147, 172
Throwing, 23, 24, 26, 28, 34, 35, 42,
    51, 66, 79, 88, 94, 129, 146, 148,
    149
Thumb, 63, 151
Tibia (shin-bone), 34
Tibial tubercle, 121

244 Index

Tibiofemoral (knee) joint, 152
Tiredness, 93
Tobogganing, 89
Toe-nails, 134
Toes, 100, 165
Tooth decay, 176
Trainability, 57
Training, 57, 60, 63–5, 76, 79, 175, 199
Training diary, 40
Training of Young Athletes Project (TOYA), 97
Training programmes, 44, 47, 59, 70, 133
Trampolining, 40, 169
'Trapped nerve(s)', 120, 146
Traumatic injuries, 116, 133, 141, 150, 152, 157, 159
Treadmill(s), 33, 55
Trendelenburg's sign, 107
Triathlon, 25, 66
Tricycle, 23
Triglycerides, 40, 197
Tripartite patella, 122
Trunk, 33, 63, 79, 87, 108, 109, 144–8, 170
'Tumble-tot' gymnastics, 23
Tumour(s), 74, 124

Ulna, 150
Ultrasound, 74, 129, 149
United States, 8, 97, 137, 194

Vaccinations, 22
Vaile, Bryn, 12–15
Valgus angle, 35
Vastus medialis muscle, 103, 142, 156, 157, 159, 166, 167, 168
Vegetarianism, 193, 201
Ventilation threshold, 57
Ventilatory equivalent, 49

Ventricular mass, 53
Vertebral column (backbone), 33, 36, 195
Vertical jump tests, 35
Viral infection, 18, 48, 93
Visco-elastic structures, 61
Vitamin supplements, 174, 193, 205
Vitamins, 59, 133, 176, 180–1, 197
VO_2 max, 54–5, 58–61, 69
Volleyball, 151, 166
Voluntary dehydration, 69

Walking, 16, 22, 39, 60, 61, 72, 90, 125, 134
Warm-down, 30, 87
Warm-up, 30, 65, 87
Water, 68, 69, 80, 89, 180, 197, 207; polo, 85; ski jumping, 146
'Weak ankles', 137
Weight, 54, 99, 194
Weight control, 182, 187, 194, 203–5
Weight training, 29, 30, 43, 53, 142, 168
Weightlifters, 123
Weightlifting, 14, 29, 41, 43, 53, 129, 146
'Whingeing child syndrome', 73
Wimbledon tennis tournament, 19
Windpipe, 81
Wingate Anaerobic Test, 45–6
Wobble board, 100, 136, 137, 166
Wound(s), 79, 120
Wrestlers, 52
Wrestling, 89, 146, 148, 208
Wrist, 36, 124, 151

X-rays, 36, 124, 125, 129, 170, 171, 173

Yoga-style stretching, 64, 147

Zinc, 192

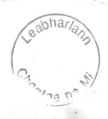